ADDITIONAL PRAISE FOR *THE CENTERED HEART*

"Beautifully written and filled with actionable information, *The Centered Heart* is required reading for anyone with a family or personal history of heart disease. This book leaves you empowered and inspired to make changes essential for both quality of life and better health outcomes."

—**Amy Rothenberg**, ND, author of *You Finished Treatment, Now What? A Field Guide for Cancer Survivors*

"An invaluable resource! From Amendola's description of her own compelling journey of self-healing through the ancient tools of yoga and Ayurveda to her incomparable experience working directly with heart patients for many decades, this book will be an invaluable resource for the practical and useful application of these research-proven tools for improving heart health and overall well-being."

—**Baxter Bell**, MD, author of *Yoga for Health Aging*

"Susi Amendola is a rare teacher and writer—one who can meet you wherever you are with the honesty, compassion, and wisdom that come from being deeply rooted in the Yoga tradition, lived experience, and current science. This beautiful, luminous book can change your life and heal your heart. It feels like an act of grace."

—**Michele Marie Desmarais**, PhD, author of *Changing Minds: Mind, Consciousness, and Identity in Patañjali's Yoga-sūtra and Cognitive Neuroscience*; associate professor of religious studies, Native American studies, and medical humanities faculty at the University of Nebraska Omaha

"A very informative book! Susi Amendola, a renowned yoga therapist, combines her wealth of expertise with a compassionate understanding of the human condition to deliver an innovative guide to heart health. I believe this book serves as a beacon of knowledge for anyone seeking a holistic approach to heart wellness. *The Centered Heart* is a vital resource, providing insights on healing, improving heart health, and achieving a better quality of life."

—**Vaidya Rajesh Kotecha**, secretary to the government of India, Ministry of Ayush; former vice chancellor, Gujarat Ayurved University; recipient of the Padma Shri from the president of India

THE CENTERED HEART

THE CENTERED HEART

Evidence–Based, Mind–Body Practices to Stress Less and Improve Cardiac Health

SUSI AMENDOLA

ROWMAN & LITTLEFIELD
Lanham • Boulder • New York • London

Published by Rowman & Littlefield
An imprint of The Rowman & Littlefield Publishing Group, Inc.
4501 Forbes Boulevard, Suite 200, Lanham, Maryland 20706
www.rowman.com

86-90 Paul Street, London EC2A 4NE

British Library Cataloguing in Publication Information Available

Library of Congress Cataloging-in-Publication Data
Names: Amendola, Susi, author.
Title: The centered heart : evidence-based, mind-body practices to stress less and improve cardiac health / Susi Amendola.
Description: Lanham : Rowman & Littlefield, 2024. | Includes bibliographical references and index.
Identifiers: LCCN 2023039133 (print) | LCCN 2023039134 (ebook) | ISBN 9781538183243 (cloth) | ISBN 9781538183250 (ebook)
Subjects: LCSH: Mind and body. | Stress management.
Classification: LCC BF151 .A45 2024 (print) | LCC BF151 (ebook) | DDC 155.9/042—dc23/eng/20231206
LC record available at https://lccn.loc.gov/2023039133
LC ebook record available at https://lccn.loc.gov/2023039134

♾️™ The paper used in this publication meets the minimum requirements of American National Standard for Information Sciences—Permanence of Paper for Printed Library Materials, ANSI/NISO Z39.48-1992.

To my dear mother, Beverly Amendola, a lifelong seeker of wisdom and truth.

Your light shines forever in my heart.

Contents

LIST OF TABLES AND FIGURES

ACKNOWLEDGMENTS

A deep bow to my teachers and mentors: Swami Rama, Swami Veda, Dr. Rolf Sovik, Pandit Rajmani Tigunait, Nischala Joy Devi, Amy Matthews, Yogacharya Dr. Ananda Balayogi Bhavanani, Dr. Rajesh Kotecha, Dr. Baxter Bell, Margot Pope, Dr. Michelle DesMarais, and so many more, some who I don't know personally but whose written and spoken words have lifted me and illuminated the path just when I needed it most. Heartfelt gratitude to the multitude of gurus and teachers who have practiced, protected, and passed on the ancient tradition of yoga, and to India for sharing it with the world.

My deep gratitude to all the Senior Trainers, Stress Management Specialists, and team members from Ornish Lifestyle Medicine. Working with you has been a delightful and gratifying ride. And to my dear friends, such gifted healers, Mimi O'Connor and Brett Kite, thank you. Working beside you for all these years has been a spiritual experience filled with love and joy.

Thank you to Dr. Dean Ornish who, as a pioneer of Lifestyle Medicine, has empowered so many individuals, giving them agency in their own healing. I am so grateful to have been given the opportunity to work with you and in your program.

Thank you to the community of students and teachers at Yoga Now Omaha. Your support and dedication have been incentives for this book.

To my beloved daughters, Terra Goulden, Grace Gillespie, Daisy Friedman, and Marissa McMillin. You each lift me up and inspire me in different ways, and I am so grateful for your wisdom and love. To your children, my grandchildren, Freya, Cosima, Jayden, and Esme, you are our future, may you lead us into a more conscious and unified world.

To my friend and sister Sandy Aquila, thank you for the beautiful headshot and for picking up your phone at all hours to just listen and offer just the right amount of guidance at just the right time. Thank you Michael Cerizo for your brilliant photographs. Thank you to all my friends and family who have offered support and insight that has found its way into this book, Michelle Miller, Liz Dolejs, Patrick Davis, Tony Hron, Jon Amendola, Jan Morgan, Frank Amendola, Dirk Gillespie, Daria Hlazatova, Jacqueline Wilber, and so many more: I beg your forgiveness for not mentioning you by name.

Thank you Rachel Lehmann Haupt at StoryMade for your early edits and encouragement. You are a wizard. Melissa Nissen (Missy), thank you beyond words for your editing and unwavering support. You are wise beyond your years, and a true healer at heart. Your buoyant cheerful nature has breathed life into this project, and I am deeply grateful.

To the team at Rowman & Littlefield for picking up this book and seeing its potential.

Lastly, to my sweetheart and husband Josh Friedman, for your tireless efforts to encourage me and help me see this project to the end, you are the embodiment of kindness and compassion. Your support, patience, and love mean the world to me. You are my second heart, and I am forever grateful to you.

Disclaimer

This book is for educational and informational purposes only and is not intended to be a substitute for the medical advice of a licensed physician. This book is intended to help encourage and empower you to connect with your own healing power and inner knowing about your body and health. Please take that knowingness with you when consulting with your doctor in any matters relating to your health.

How to Use the Practices Offered in this Book

The practices in this book can be read aloud by teachers to students, health-care practitioners to patients, therapists to clients, parents to children, and yoga teachers to yoga students, or they can be spoken into a recording device and played back for you, your family, or your friends as needed.

Be creative and enjoy.

Please scan the above QR code with the camera on your phone or tablet, or visit www.yourcenteredheart.com to access audio practices from this book, read by the author.

Bonus materials are included.

Introduction

WHEN I GREW UP IN THE SUBURBS OF CHICAGO, I LOVED TO PLAY in nature. I had a treehouse, collected worms after it rained, made necklaces out of hollyhock seeds, and nursed sick baby birds. Often, I would lie in the grass and watch the clouds, and during those moments I always felt the presence of something much greater than myself. By the time I reached my teens, I was a fun-loving extrovert—creative, spiritual, empathetic, and joyful.

And then one summer when I was sixteen, something shifted dramatically. I had an unexpected reaction after smoking pot at a party with friends, which set into motion a pattern of anxiety and depression that lingered for years and changed me forever. Was the pot laced? Was I allergic? A hormonal coincidence? Did it loosen a pattern of anxiety that had been deep and unexpressed until then? None of that is completely clear even now. It was as if my nervous system was short-circuited and my old way of being completely dismantled. I felt like I was trapped inside myself looking through a haze that couldn't be lifted. Everything I did made me panic. I was afraid to leave my house, go to school, drive a car, wake up in the morning, and go to sleep at night.

Overwhelmed, and unable to pull myself up, I sank deeper into depression. I hid my suffering and was too afraid and ashamed to talk about it, for fear no one would understand. The doctors I saw threw their hands up with nothing to offer. Mental health treatments in the late 1970s in the Midwest were mostly unrefined. I imagined the diagnosis for anxiety would be something out of the movie *One Flew Over the Cuckoo's Nest*. A doctor would say, "You had a nervous breakdown." This would be followed by a month or more stay in the mental hospital, and drug and electric shock therapy that did more harm than good. I had witnessed this with family friends, and I wanted no part of a treatment plan like that. And so without a path to healing, anxiety and panic robbed me of much of my teenage years. My family and friends chalked it up to a period of moodiness and teenage angst, while I wandered alone in the darkness looking for anything that could relieve my suffering.

In the midst of this period, my mom connected with one of the first swamis to come to this country from India. As yoga was beginning to make its debut in the States, Elmer and Alyce Green, the scientific founders of the Menninger Foundation, known for their psychotherapeutic approach to mental health, which at the time was innovative and provocative, had the idea to conduct one of the first Western scientific studies of this swami's abilities as a yogi.[1] They had a well-equipped laboratory designed to investigate voluntary control of psychophysiological processes. During their studies, they found he could move a knitting needle with his mind, put his heart into fibrillation, and recount conversations from another room while he was actually in deep sleep (yoga nidra).

The more recent understanding of neuroscience and the impact of brain-body connection was not yet an idea, but the Menninger Foundation and the swami wanted to document the scientific understanding of Yoga. These studies helped establish yoga in the West and pointed to the powerful effects these practices could have on physical, mental, and emotional health and well-being. Today, these practices are now well-proven in many contemporary neuroscience studies of "mindfulness," and increasingly in yoga therapy.

Soon, this swami opened an ashram in the suburbs of Chicago where hundreds of people would come to hear him speak and teach on the ancient tradition of yoga. The ashram evolved into one of the first holistic clinics where his students, who were mostly medical doctors, psychologists, and other health professionals, came to teach yoga and practice what is now known as holistic health, or "lifestyle medicine," an emerging field where the emphasis is placed on diet, exercise, and stress management as a path to healing.

My mom, with five kids at home, four of which were in high school, had started doing yoga to manage her own stress. One day she invited me to go with her to visit the center to take classes and meet the swami. We argued most of the way there. I'm not even sure why. Maybe because I was a teenager and that's what teenage girls and mothers do, but when we arrived at the clinic, my mood changed. It was a simple and peaceful place—a small campus with just three buildings tucked off the main road lined with trees and beautiful gardens. People were walking on the grounds in flowing white cotton yoga clothes, and the fragrance of Indian spices and incense hung in the air.

As we walked up the path to the main building together, I felt immediately drawn to the swami, a statuesque figure in long robes standing at the front door. Greeting us at the door, he pulled me into what felt like a familiar and loving embrace. "Hey kid, I've been waiting for you," he said in a commanding voice. He then looked at my mom and like a scolding father added, "Be nice to your daughter, don't fight with her, she's a good kid." And with a childlike grin, he whispered in my ear, "and you should listen to your mother." Wait. How did he know we were fighting in the car? She hadn't had time to tell him that. But the answer didn't matter to me. Instead, I was just relieved that I felt seen and understood. He was clearly advocating for me.

As the crowd gathered around the swami, he was shuffled into a big lecture hall where he spoke to a large group of followers in his thick Indian accent. I found myself hanging on his every word. I felt like he was talking directly to me. There was hope, love, and unity in his message, and he felt as deep as the ocean and as big as the universe. Tears were welling up from a place inside of me that knew the truth and wanted more. No one I had ever seen or heard had grabbed my heart and soul in this way.

Before we left, I looked at him from across the room and noticed his skin was shining with what looked like a radiant blue tint to it. I asked my mom why his skin looked so blue. She turned with a puzzled look but never answered. It wasn't until years later that I realized that many Indian saints and sages are depicted with blue skin because blue, the color of the sky and the ocean, is symbolic of the infinite.

Over the next several months, I spent more and more time taking yoga and meditation classes at the clinic, listening to the swami speak, and practicing yoga while meditating on my own at home. The center became my refuge. Slowly, I noticed things starting to change. I began to find my way out of the crippling anxiety that had stolen the person I used to be.

After a short time, I decided to move to Pennsylvania, where the swami had set up a new institute for the study of yoga. It was a lot like an ashram but more Americanized and research based. The swami wanted yoga to have its rightful place in the world of science. An ashram, with its spiritual focus, would perhaps be viewed as irrelevant to the world of research and science, so students were encouraged to dress in a modest but familiar way, while merging the Indian practices and traditions with American culture.

I became a resident there and worked for my stay as a cook in the yogic/Ayurvedic kitchen where we prepared vegetarian meals for all the residents and guests. A yogic kitchen is one where the food is light and fresh to support the internal practices of yoga. The food is prepared with love according to the seasons, borrowing from the principles of Ayurveda, the sister science of yoga. Ayurveda uses the knowledge of the elements and the six tastes principle to use food as medicine. There is an art and a science to this style of cooking, and I was both in training and training others. I also spent time working with children at the institute's Montessori school while attending daily classes in yoga, meditation, and philosophy. I took workshops in all kinds of health-related topics, ate vegetarian meals, and walked outside in the fresh, open mountain air. The structure, the food, the yoga practices, the sense of community, and living in nature became the foundation and the foothold I needed to find my way back to myself, the self I knew before anxiety had taken hold of me.

I stayed there for almost five years. I met my husband, fell in love, and got married. He was "a boy from Nebraska" (as the swami called him) who was open-minded, creative, and curious. He had met the swami at a gathering at the University of Nebraska-Lincoln and was so taken by him that he followed him to Pennsylvania. Soon after we were married, we had our first daughter. Young couples and families were springing up everywhere. The place seemed magical, and our lives felt deeply meaningful with the support of this close-knit community.

After several years of study, work, devotion, and practice, stories of sexual abuse by the swami began to circulate. My husband and I, both disoriented and disillusioned, decided to leave the institute with our young daughter in tow, to start over in his hometown of Omaha, Nebraska. I was devastated to leave the community. The anxiety and depression that I had worked so hard to overcome began slowly creeping back. With a sadness that settled in my heart and lungs, I landed in the hospital close to death with advanced pneumonia. When I recovered, my symptoms of panic returned, and my climb out, while not unfamiliar, seemed insurmountable.

Yoga practice became more important to me as the question of its validity in the face of this flawed guru haunted me. The teaching that was clear now was to find my own innate wisdom, my own inner teacher. Yoga was all I knew and all I had. With a tried-and-true belief that a yoga practice could help my body, heart, and mind, I returned to my own practices, and I opened The Omaha Yoga & Bodywork Center, one of the first and oldest yoga centers in the Midwest. Over the years, I created programs to train yoga teachers, sponsor well-known speakers on yoga, and bring the healing practices of yoga to businesses, schools, and the community. Currently called Yoga Now, it has been a stronghold in the community for over forty years. As I helped others with the practices that turned my own life around, their stories of health and healing have served as inspiration for my own.

In the fall of 1992, I got a call that changed the direction of my life and work. Dr. Dean Ornish, an emerging leader in the field of lifestyle medicine, was piloting a study in Omaha (with Mutual of Omaha) that involved reversing heart disease without drugs or surgery. The intervention consisted of lifestyle changes that included a low-fat vegetarian diet, moderate exercise, group support, and yoga as stress management. He had done an initial study that included a small sample of participants with some positive and encouraging results.[2] Now he was looking to do a multi-center lifestyle trial with the hope of replicating outcomes with a much wider population.

The hospital called me looking for a yoga teacher for the study. They wanted one with training in relaxation, meditation, breathing, yoga postures, and yoga philosophy. Essentially, someone with experience in using yoga for healing. It was as if they had written the description with me in mind. I would be part of a transdisciplinary team, working side by side with medical doctors, dietitians, and mental health practitioners.

While this looked like a dream job, I was also torn internally. Modern medicine supports an external locus of control, a belief that healing happens outside of us. The doctors heal you, the medicines will make you well, the surgeries will fix you. Yoga, on the other hand, supports an internal locus of control, including self-responsibility, self-care, and self-healing. While this type of healing may also involve some interventions from outside, the individual who is practicing is the most important part of the equation. How would I navigate this profound philosophical difference? Was there really a way to bring those two seemingly opposing views of healing together? Because this program would take place in a hospital setting, would the singular influence of a Western medicine approach to healing overshadow the deeper and more comprehensive approach to healing that I knew yoga embraces? Would the use of yoga in this program be able to maintain its integrity and depth, or would it be watered down to fit a more Western medical model of healing?

With all these questions and my own anxiety still looming, my first answer to the request was an emphatic NO. Yet, I knew the power of yoga in my own healing journey could help me serve others. In the tradition of yoga, they say that your dharma, or life work, is "doing what's yours to do, based on your gifts, your nature, and your strengths." I knew this was mine to do, my calling, my dharma. After all, heart disease was rampant in my own Italian family. Could I really pass on the opportunity to be part of a healing community and the introduction of yoga into the world of medicine? My second answer was YES.

The lifestyle program started in the hospital in 1993 with a cohort of no more than fifteen participants who would spend four hours together two times a week. In that time they exercised together, talked about their feelings in a group, ate a low-fat vegetarian meal, and practiced stress management (yoga). My role as the "Stress Management Specialist" was not only to teach them yoga techniques but to help them develop a sense of empowerment around their own healing and home practice. I spent just one hour with them during stress management, but they were expected to practice at home for a minimum of one hour a day, every day, on their own.

These were not people who chose to practice yoga. These were people who wanted to get better, and their doctors were urging them to try this new program. In some cases, they had already had more than one surgery and were out of options. In other cases, they were trying to avoid a new surgery.

Yoga was foreign to almost all of them, and my job was to find ways to adapt the practices and support them in all the lifestyle changes. Based on my own history, I understood their desperation, and I knew those feelings of hopelessness, fear, and anxiety. I felt a kinship as we started the journey together. Their honesty, determination, hope, and willingness became my motivation. In one of our first cohorts, I worked with someone who was put in our program while waiting for a heart transplant, and I watched him come off the transplant list in just twelve weeks of doing the protocols. Another man, who had such severe angina he couldn't walk across the room without having to sit down, started to hike. Several patients came off their heart medications, while others with type II diabetes reduced and even stopped their insulin. I couldn't believe what I was seeing firsthand. The changes were undeniable.

After the first year, Mutual of Omaha noted an insurance savings of almost $30,000 per patient in the first year.[3] The stories of restored health and hope were rolling in. The study was then replicated at several sites across the country with the same results. For the next twelve years, I would work with Dean and his team to refine and deliver the program in a hospital setting.

My work both with this program and in my own private practice has gifted me the opportunity to hold the hearts of so many, supporting them in those tender, sacred moments of extreme vulnerability that we all face at one time or another in our lives. I now know that it's in these moments when we often meet our true selves. When suffering or loss comes, and the ground we were standing on becomes shaky or nonexistent, we begin to search for help and answers. It's here in this moment of questioning, searching, and uncertainty that space opens and the things that matter most become clear. We come face-to-face with the stripped-down version of ourselves. There is nothing to prove, nowhere to run, and nothing to hide. It's in that moment that a healing shift is possible. It's in that moment that everything can change.

Through my experience teaching yoga in a medical setting, I have discovered new gems of knowledge from a wisdom tradition delivered from teacher to student, generation to generation, for centuries. Their value, insight, and merits have been proven repeatedly. Most importantly, these practices have been validated by practitioners who have done the practices and reaped the benefits in their own lives. And now their efficacy has been tested and researched in many peer-reviewed journals.

This book is the culmination of what I have compiled through my suffering, my studies, and ultimately my own triumph in my journey back to health. It is what I have learned through the authenticity and openness that others have shared with me during their own sojourn to healing. May this be an inspiration and a blessing. May this book illuminate a path that leads you back to health, back to yourself, and back to your own centered heart.

Uncovering the Calm Within

"When we are no longer able to change a situation, we are challenged to change ourselves."

—VICTOR FRANKL[1]

SCENARIO 1

It's Monday morning and you wake up to the loud beeping of your alarm. Groggy and unfocused, you grab a coffee and get ready for work. Your mind is still racing after a rather stressful night of worry about a meeting you feel unprepared to handle. You spent most of the night tossing and turning, rather than sleeping. As you get in the car, you turn on the morning news and feel agitation and anxiety. You arrive at work with little time to spare before your dreaded meeting. It's the beginning of your day, and you are already feeling exhausted and overwhelmed. During the day, you find yourself on edge, off-center, and ineffective. The meeting didn't go well. At some point you realize you haven't even taken a deep breath and your shoulders are so tense they are squeezed up around your ears as your day jumps from one emergency to the next. By the time you get home, you can't even think about cooking, exercise, or relaxation. You plop down in front of your screen and watch the news, scroll through social media until, with little or no energy left for yourself, you grab whatever food is easy and you proceed to overeat. By bedtime you find it hard to settle down. The day's events are still percolating, and you are concerned you may have another sleepless night ahead.

These moments of stress often define us.

SCENARIO 2

You wake up 30 minutes earlier than usual to the soothing music you programmed for your alarm. You want to sleep in, but you know these 30 minutes will give you more rest and peace than the sleep you are missing. You sit up and do some deep breathing and meditation to center yourself before the day begins. At the end of the practices, you use imagery to see yourself staying present and centered throughout the day. Before you leave for work, you sit down to some fresh berries and warm tea. Using mindful eating skills, you connect with your food in a way that helps you feel nourished and calm.

Once in the car you begin to set some intentions for your day. Rather than reaching for the radio dial or your podcasts, you imagine yourself moving through your day with ease and grace. You arrive at your desk feeling centered and prepared. As you find yourself meeting the challenges of the day, you return to some slow deep breaths and come back to that early morning experience of being deeply relaxed and focused. As the day unfolds, you feel the familiar rise of your shoulders next to your ears. You take a moment to do a few gentle stretches at your desk. You lift and lower your shoulders and use some of your gentle neck and shoulder movements to tune into your body and release any collected tension. As stressful situations arise, you reconnect with your set intentions for the day, and they help reframe your experience.

At the end of the day you feel tired, but you are not exhausted. Once you arrive home, you do a few gentle movements to release any tension in the body, followed by some breathing exercises and meditation. Now you are ready to start your evening. You might take a walk or find the food that you prepared over the weekend and heat it up. You don't feel the need to overeat now that you are more relaxed and present. Now you feel the space and ease to do those creative projects or read your favorite book, or even connect with friends or loved ones. The difference in how you feel today is in stark contrast to your usual feelings of overwhelm and exhaustion. When you go to bed you listen to a systematic relaxation practice, and you drift into a deep and restful sleep.

If you are living in Scenario 1, this new path in Scenario 2 may sound ridiculous and impossible. However, deep within each of us is the calm we long for, the calm that can carry us through times of uncertainty, and the calm we need to recharge and heal. The practices outlined in this book are designed to help you uncover that calm, stress less, and recover your health. With time and dedicated practice, Scenario 2 may begin to feel within your reach, and you will start to notice changes you hadn't thought were possible.

We are all living somewhere in the space between ease and dis-ease, and the choices we make each day about how we live can move us closer to one end or the other on that continuum of health. Stress is itself an epidemic of monumental proportions, and the way that we react and respond to stressful situations plays a major role in our suffering. The CDC notes that 75 to 90 percent of all doctor's office visits are for stress-related ailments and complaints. Additionally, the medical establishment has long confirmed the link between stress and heart disease, which is the number one cause of death, with approximately one person dying every thirty-six seconds in the United States from cardiovascular disease (that's one in every four deaths).[2] We never think it will be us who will be affected. We make excuses and pretend everything is fine.

Prioritizing stress management practices in your life makes you feel in control and at ease. You have more space, feel more joy, and find yourself responding differently to those everyday stressors. Things that used to bother you don't seem to bother you in the same way. You can create a different way of being with just a few simple practices. A way of being that, in time, changes the course of your life and health.

Living in a way that is more connected to an inner calm is a vital part of self-care, yet often we look at self-care as selfish or overindulgent. That's because we are rewarded for overworking and for being *stressed out*, as if it were a badge of honor that you have earned through your neglect of yourself and ignoring your own needs. Yet no one ever says, "Hey, keep up the good work that led to the heart attack you just had!" or "Congrats, your blood pressure is up; you've really outdone yourself!" or "Wonderful news about your adrenal exhaustion! I can see you're really giving it your all these days!"

Obviously, self-blame for these choices is not the answer. Instead, it's about redirecting your energies into what you can do to stay healthy without retreating to a monastery, an ashram, or an organic farm in the country. How we react and respond to every-day stressors can be the difference between health and disease. Talk therapies and didactic classes on stress management seem like they will relieve our suffering, but they alone don't really do the trick because stress and trauma find their way into our bodies. We need therapies that address the body *and* the mind, therapies that bring us back to ourselves.

Studies are now revealing that somatic therapies, which are defined as therapies that target the mind and body, reduce stress and stress-related illness. The word *somatic* comes from the root *soma*, meaning "of the body," and these practices serve to bring you into a relationship with your own body. When we experience stress or trauma, we tend to move out of the body so we don't have to feel the discomfort. We may find ourselves unable to feel a sense of residency in our own bodies, setting up a disconnection between the body and the mind. It's almost as if we begin to leave ourselves when there is a painful or difficult situation or expe-rience. That disconnection removes us from the innate wisdom of the body. It leaves us without the resource of our own inner wisdom and knowingness.

Practices like yoga can return us, bring us back into listening to that wisdom, back into balance so healing can occur. Yoga is a somatic practice, but often it is offered and practiced in a way that doesn't lead to embodiment. Doing yoga like a game of "Simon Says" is not somatic, but when we shift from thinking and doing to feeling and being, we are practicing in a somatic way. Yoga doesn't make stress go away, but it gives us a healthy way of dealing with it. A large study investigating the link between psychological stress and cardiovascular disease (CVD) found that the effects of acute versus long-term stressors on cardiac functioning were determined by the coping strategies used.[3] These strategies played a major role in determining the impact of all stressors, highlighting the need to properly cope with the stress that we have in our lives, rather than simply looking to reduce stressors. Coping strategies like those found in the ancient and traditional practices of yoga, such as gentle movements, breathing, relaxation, meditation, and imagery, offer hope and help.

The effectiveness of yoga in reducing risk factors for CVD and other stress-related, lifestyle illnesses is well established in scientific research.[4] In a 2019 comprehensive analysis of 149 publications on yoga and cardiovascular health, of which 44 percent were clinical trials, the authors noted that pharmacological treatment alone may not be a cure-all for such diseases, since the treatments may cause side effects, and may not be effective in healing CVD.[5] Fortunately, yoga that is supplemented with other healthy lifestyle and stress management techniques such as diet, exercise, and visualization is becoming more widely recommended by doctors for heart patients to lower patients' dependence on pharmacological treatment and to decrease the risk of adverse effects.

In a research review looking at the role of yoga in the prevention and management of lifestyle disorders, a friend and colleague,
Dr. Ananda Balayogi Bhavanani, states:

> Comprehensive reviews have suggested that yoga reduces the
> cardiovascular risk profile by decreasing the "fight or flight"
> response by modulating the adrenal glands production of cor-
> tisol and adrenaline. It also promotes a feeling of well-being
> by enhancing parasympathetic activity known as the relaxation
> response.[6]

Dr. Bhavanani also notes that yoga may have a positive influence
in just a single session. His research team looked at 1,896 normal
individuals as well as patients with different medical conditions
and found a healthy reduction in heart rate, blood pressure, and
cardiac risk factors following a single yogic session.[7]

Health and healing come from a state of harmony, unity, and
calm awareness. Yet somehow, we have gotten the message that
it's a state we need to achieve, or something we acquire from outside of us. We push ourselves in hopes of becoming more healthy
and more fit. We measure health by the number of minutes we
walk, how many calories we eat, how much weight we lift, how
long we meditate. We think that the more we can squeeze into our
routine the healthier we will be. We are missing the point.

The essence of health is deep within each of us. Yoga provides
a compass for developing an internal locus of control, finding
balance and calm within. Health stems from this internal state
of harmony and self-responsibility. A doctor can tell us we are
healthy, but if we don't feel good, is that really health? Yoga
defines health as ease. Do I feel at ease in my own body, mind,
and heart? Our health is determined by our internal experience,
not an external measure.

The somatic practices of yoga can help you not only tune
into how you are feeling, but also provide tools and practices that

return you to a state of balance and ease so healing can occur. Relaxing the body, steadying the breath, quieting the mind and heart—all return us to a sense of inner peace and ease.

Think of it as an awakening of your own personal power to affect your well-being. This power is far greater than you ever realized. Each chapter contained in this book is an introduction and immersion into one aspect of these practices that is healing: postures, breathing, relaxation, meditation, imagery, compassion, and connection to nature. The chapters are then woven together with stories from my students and heart patients, and with practices that provide a map to self-discovery and self-healing. Included are details of how to choose and shape each practice to make it personal and relevant, as well as the science that supports why the practice will help you reclaim your health and uncover the calm within.

Gentle Movements

Deep Listening

"Your body is your best guide. It constantly tells you, in the form of pain or sensations, what's working for you and what's not."

—HINA HASHMI[1]

A CENTERING MOMENT

Imagine the Weight of the World Rolling Off Your Shoulders

- Sit or stand comfortably.
- Take a conscious slow, deep breath.
- Now as you inhale, lift and squeeze both shoulders.
- Hold them and squeeze even more.
- As you exhale, lower the shoulders with an audible sigh through the mouth.
- Imagine the weight of the world rolling off your shoulders.

- Allow any tension to exit through the fingertips.
- Repeat 3 times and then roll your shoulders, soften, be still, and listen.

Much of our time is spent paying attention to what's outside of us. We keep ourselves so busy that we rarely take a moment to check in with how we are feeling, not to mention take time to listen to what our bodies might be telling us about ourselves. Sadly, it often takes some kind of illness or incident for us to slow down and drop in.

When my daughter was young, she used to complain of headaches while she was in school. I would say to her, "Gracie, is there something you're doing with your body that may be causing this? Are you squinting to see the board, or holding your head in some way that may be causing your neck or shoulders to tense up? Maybe you could pay attention to how you are sitting or moving to get some answers." She looked at me with a blank stare and said, "Mom, I have no idea what is happening inside my body when I am in school. I am listening to the teacher and doing what she tells me. That's all. I don't have time to pay attention to my body." There you have it. We are trained from a very young age that what is important is *outside* of us. The information our body is offering us is not as important as what is being offered outside of ourselves. We are taught to overlook our own inner wisdom and ignore the signals that may be a cautionary tale about our own health.

One way to tune into that inner wisdom is through the practice of postures. Postures, or gentle movements, are a way to embody awareness. Ancient Indian medicine says, "Disease knocks three times, and if you don't listen, it takes you." Practicing postures allows you to move into the spaces of your own body and listen to the information the body is offering you about yourself. So many people have said to me after a serious health incident, "I knew there was something wrong, I just didn't listen." *Postures help you listen.* They return your awareness to those spaces you have left or ignored due to trauma, stress, or illness. And while postures also build strength, flexibility, and balance, most importantly they allow you to drop in, listen closely, and reclaim the spaces of your own body. In this process, you become more attuned to yourself and are better able to make choices that support your health and well-being.

The body reflects the habitual, not the occasional. What we do, how we think, and how we move are all subject to our habits. When we repeat a movement over and over, it has an effect on us. It's like placing a stone in a stream. If you keep placing stones in the same place over and over, the stream eventually changes its direction. The process is much the same when we move the body in the same way over and over, for better or for worse. The postures, or poses, outlined in this chapter are meant to increase or even shift the flow of blood and energy, opening areas that have been blocked through held tension or trauma. Over time, and with gentleness, a new pathway opens, and a new habit is formed.

When practicing postures, it is important to develop a sense of curiosity. If you only do the movements with a goal of getting them "right," you will surely miss the point. I have been to many yoga or movement classes where it feels like a game of "Simon Says." The teacher shouts out a command and everyone follows along. In this practice, following along is only helpful in the beginning until the positions feel more natural. With repetition you will begin to remember the movements, and once they are familiar, they can be done with an internal focus and a sense of inquisitiveness. This helps foster the kind of interest that invites you into a new way of seeing and being.

While exploring your edges and boundaries during these movements, you might ask yourself, "Am I comfortable here?" or "Where am I holding on?" or "Could I soften anything I don't need to maintain this posture?" or "What thoughts or feelings am I having?" The questioning here is not for the sake of analyzing or judging. This kind of inquiry can help uncover the source of discomfort and bring you into a more connected relationship with your own body.

In life we are constantly analyzing and judging our experiences as a way to make sense of things on an intellectual level, but in this practice, we are asked to set aside judging and analyzing and become more of a witness to our experience. We try to observe the mental chatter without labels or judgments, without analyzing or ruminating, and without getting lost in our stories. We start to let go of our inclination to compete with ourselves, beat ourselves up, or even praise ourselves. Essentially, we step out of our own way and try to cultivate a fresh perspective. We create space for our bodies to teach us through experience.

There has been some rather significant research done on individual practices and the benefits from doing a yoga session that includes postures and breathing. A study completed at the Center for Yoga Therapy and Research and published in the journal *Alternative & Integrative Medicine* showed that when participants performed postures and breathing practices, statistically significant reductions in all the studied cardiovascular parameters were observed. The magnitude of reductions was more significant in those with hypertension and cardiovascular disease.[2] Another study published in the journal *Biological Research for Nursing* showed that the somatic practices of yoga have been effective in reducing stress and inflammatory biomarkers. This study showed that these practices not only impact heart disease but can reduce inflammation that is often at the root of heart disease and other chronic conditions.[3]

It is incredible that we now have the technology to measure the health benefits of yoga to ensure that these practices are effective, but yoga is an ancient philosophy and practice that has been done for thousands of years. It is a lineage of peace and healing that cannot always be measured and quantified, but rather, it can be felt and known through personal experience. This serves as a reminder to trust your own felt experience as you practice.

SO NOW WE BEGIN YOGA

Within this chapter you will find a basic routine of specific postures to increase self-awareness and support the heart and healing. Each posture can be done to suit each individual's needs and conditions. The practices are designed to help you develop a sense of attunement with your own body while experiencing a greater sense of freedom, flow, and ease.

In my own experience, I have seen firsthand the impact of this simple yet very effective posture series. I have watched people come into a session with what looks like the weight of the world on their shoulders and leave feeling freer, calmer, happier, and lighter.

This gentle series, while adapted from the teachings of Swami Satchidananda and Integral Yoga, has been modified to suit the specific needs of a wide variety of abilities.[4] Always remember to honor your own body and its individual capacities and limits. The postures are meant to be practiced all together for best results, but when looking for a quick reset, they can be used individually as a 3- to 5-minute reboot.

Setting Up a Space for Practice

When setting up a space to practice, it's important to think about what will inspire you to make this practice and your body a priority. What will lift you up and encourage you to make time for yourself? We are all creatures of habit, and if we put some intentionality to our routines they can support and even heal us. Creating healthy habits takes conscious effort, but in time they become effortless.

There is a practice in yoga called Japa-Ajapa, which is the practice of repeating a mantra over and over again. It's often done with mala beads as a way to keep track of the repetitions. With practice it becomes so ingrained that when you stop, you can hear the mantra without having to say it. This is what we are doing when we show up over and over again to practice. The practice becomes an effortless habit. Simply put, if you want to have a regular practice you have to practice regularly.

By showing up over and over again, you don't have to work so hard at showing up. It becomes a routine. I often tell people, "Don't try to fit stress management practices into your life, *let your life organize around your stress management practices.*" This kind of thinking helps you make your practice a priority.

Choosing a Place to Practice

You may notice that when you pass by your kitchen, you think, "I could really use a snack right now," or when you walk past your bedroom, you might say to yourself, "Taking a nap would feel great in this moment." This is because we have trained ourselves to respond in this way by doing the same thing, in the same space, over and over again. Now the space holds that energy and calls out to you when you walk by it. This is how habits are formed.

It's helpful to pick a place in your house that feels airy, spacious, light, and calm. Not everyone has the option of picking a separate room in their living space, so carving out a place in your favorite room can work as well. Some people may even choose to do the practices in their own bed, so they don't have to get up and down from the floor. Others may choose to use a chair to sit in. I've included practices that can be done on the floor, in bed, or seated in a chair.

Choosing a Time to Practice

When choosing a time to practice, you may want to consider a time of day that works best for you and your lifestyle. Carve out a time when you can be regular and honor the time each day for your self-care. Choose a time when you will be undisturbed, so you can settle into yourself. Some people like the early morning because they feel fresh. Working with the body first thing can help bring awareness to your body and prepare you for the activities of the day with energy and presence. Remember that if you practice in the morning, the body may be a little stiffer, so be gentle and go slow.

Others like to practice in the evening after the day is done and they can settle into themselves and transition from all the happenings of the day. At the end of the day, the body is a little more flexible and movements may flow with greater ease and grace. It is always best to practice on an empty stomach, but I find that having some tea and a small bite can take the edge off, so my stomach isn't growling.

Starting Your Practice
Now that you know where you will practice and when, start by gathering a few items:

- One or two chairs (folding chairs work well)
- Two bed pillows
- One blanket
- A yoga mat or pad (optional)

As you begin the warmups below, it is always nice to remind yourself of these notes:

- Move slowly and with awareness.
- Allow the breath to flow naturally and through the nose whenever possible.
- Breathe smoothly without holding or straining your breath.
- Start to identify your edges and pause in that place of comfort/discomfort; allow yourself to settle in.
- When you can, relax your effort.
- If you have done too much or gone too far, try doing less.
- Rest and observe when you finish. Know that the time between the poses is as important as the poses themselves.

- It can be helpful to imagine yourself doing the pose first without moving, and then practice what you imagined.

WARMUP PRACTICES

- Neck
- Shoulders
- Hands and Wrists
- Ankles and Feet

Benefits: These movements articulate the joints while delivering synovial fluid to them. They also encourage movement of blood, lymph and energy to the fingers, toes, shoulders, ankles, and neck. This can reduce the likelihood of injury and increase the ease of movement in the body.

Note: The warmups can be used as a stand-alone practice when you need them. If you have undergone a recent injury, illness, or surgery, you can use the ones that feel good to you rather than trying to do all the postures. Some days you might ask yourself, "What one or two warmups do I need today?" and listen to your own body for guidance. These warmups are simple, but powerful. Their effects on health and awareness should not be underestimated. As you pause between the movements, notice the echoes and ripples of movement in your own body.

The Practice of the Neck Exercises

- Sit in a chair or on the floor. Find the connection of your sit bones to the chair/earth.

- Begin to imagine the effortless lift of your spine up out of the pelvis into the airspace above you.

- As you exhale, lower the chin toward the chest. Keep breathing.

- Notice the stretch in the back of the neck, and observe how far down the spine you feel the stretch.

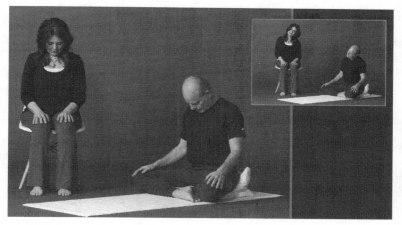

Figure 2.1. Neck Exercises.

- Slowly, on an inhale return the chin to center, and on an exhale relax.

- Inhale again and as you exhale, take the left ear toward the left shoulder. Keep the breath flowing and you notice the stretch on the side of the neck.

- As you inhale, return the head to center and relax.

- Inhale again and as you exhale, take the right ear toward the right shoulder; let the breath flow.

- As you inhale, return to center and observe. Listen and be still.

Note: *If coordinating breath and movement is confusing, just allow yourself to breathe naturally and move at your own pace.*

The Practice of the Shoulder Exercises

- Sit in a chair or on the floor.

- Inhale and gently squeeze the shoulders up next to the ears, and as you exhale, lower them, sigh, and relax.

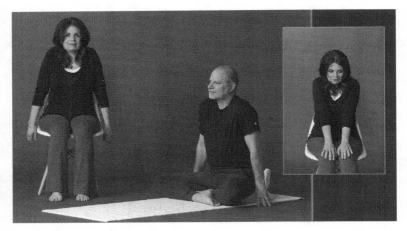

Figure 2.2. Shoulder Exercises.

- Now inhale and squeeze the shoulders together behind you. With an exhale, sigh and relax.
- Lastly, inhale and squeeze the shoulders together in front of you, and as you exhale, sigh and relax.
- Now roll both shoulders in one direction 3–5 times and then in the opposite direction 3–5 times.
- Keep the breath and movement flowing.
- When you finish, return to center and relax.

The Practice of the Hand and Wrist Exercises

- Sit in a chair or on the floor.
- Let your hands hang down alongside the body (if sitting on the floor you can also take them out in front of you).
- Open and squeeze the fingers several times.
- With the hands in loose fists, rotate the wrists slowly in one direction and then the other.
- Now shake the hands and fingers gently up and down and sideways. Turn the palms up and shake gently again.

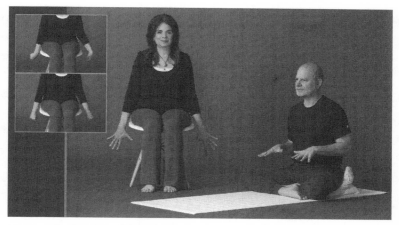

Figure 2.3. Hand and Wrist Exercises.

- Rest the hands in your lap, close the eyes, and be still.

The Practice of Ankle and Feet Exercises

- Sit in a chair or on the floor.

- Stretch your legs out in front of you and place your heels on the floor.

- Begin by pointing the toes and then flexing the feet. Repeat this 3–5 times.

- Now open and squeeze the toes several times. See if you can create some space between your toes when you open them. If some of your toes don't open, know that over time it is possible that the signal from your brain will make it to your feet and they will start to cooperate, so don't lose hope, gently keep trying.

- Rotate the ankles in one direction and then the other, making circles with the toes.

- Return to center, close your eyes, and notice the effects of the practice.

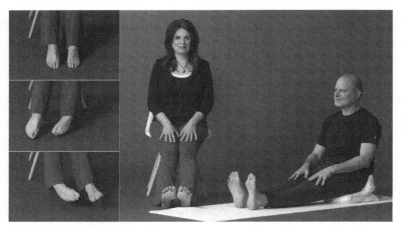

Figure 2.4. Ankle and Feet Exercises.

THE POSTURES

- Crocodile
- Cobra
- Half locust
- Seated forward bend
- Seated spinal twist
- Modified shoulder stand
- Fish

Crocodile

Crocodile pose supports resting and grounding. It is an excellent position for strengthening the diaphragm muscle, which is one of the most important muscles in the body because it facilitates deep breathing. With the face down, the mind and sense organs are turned inward and allowed to rest. This is an effective way to bring awareness to both long breathing (abdominal breathing), wide breathing (diapragmatic/ribcage breathing), and deep breathing (chest breathing). When you roll over, there is an easy transition into three-part breathing, also known as the complete yogic breath (chapter 4).

This is also a great resting position between the cobra and the half locust pose (described later). This pose also supports the natural curve of the low back. If there is discomfort from too much curve, you can place a bed pillow under your abdomen to lessen the curve and rest the back.

Benefits: Crocodile strengthens the diaphragm muscle and promotes diaphragmatic breathing. This pose increases lung capacity, stimulates the stomach and digestion, calms the nervous system, and quiets the mind.

Contraindications: If you have an abdominal aortic aneurysm or mobility issues, practice crocodile by using the chair version with your hands placed on the diaphragm.

The Practice of Crocodile on the Floor

- Lie on the floor on your stomach.

- Fold your arms and rest your forehead on your forearms. If you prefer, you can rest your cheek on your forearms.

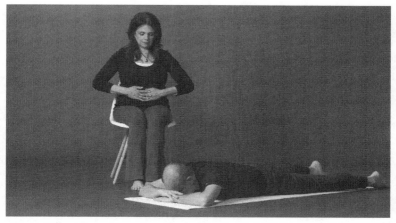

Figure 2.5. Crocodile.

- Breathe slowly and smoothly with a focus on your diaphragm muscle, which is just above your navel and just below your ribs. You can adjust your arms in or out to put the appropriate pressure on your diaphragm.

- Imagine your ribs expanding when you inhale and contracting when you exhale.

- Take several conscious, slow, deep breaths and then let your awareness and breath settle in the back side of your own heart.

- Breathe as if the back of your heart is breathing.

- Stay for several breaths and then release and roll over.

- Be still and listen.

The Practice of Crocodile in a Chair

While the benefits are a bit different when sitting up on a chair, since there is less pressure on the diaphragm, there is benefit to turning your awareness to the diaphragm muscle.

- Sit comfortably in a chair and place your hands over your diaphragm muscle just below your ribs and just above your navel.

- Apply a little pressure and imagine breathing into your hands as you inhale slowly, smoothly, and deeply.

- Take several breaths as you close your eyes and relax your shoulders.

- Release your hands from your diaphragm and place both palms briefly against your forehead. Use just a little pressure and take a couple breaths.

- Release your hands and place them in your lap.

- Notice how you feel and be still for a moment.

Cobra

It's not uncommon to experience tense, tight, and painful shoulders from trying to protect the heart both physically and emotionally. This pattern may even start to affect the upper spine from holding the shoulders forward. Doing the cobra posture regularly starts to retrain and reverse this habit. It lets the blood and energy flow freely from the heart through the shoulders and down the arms to the hands. The arms carry the action of the heart into the world, allowing us to give and receive love. Regular practice starts to open that energetic pathway.

As we begin the practice of cobra, we start by lying down on the floor, with the head turned to one side, the arms resting alongside the body. This allows the shoulder wings to relax and separate while the back of the heart becomes more exposed, bringing to awareness those emotions that we may have tucked away from ourselves. It's here we can practice holding our feelings compassionately as we observe them arising and then dissipating. We simply bear witness to whatever bubbles up in our awareness. In this way we gain the ability to sit with our difficult emotions without judging.

In the second part of cobra, we begin to lift and lengthen. The palms of the hands are planted on the floor, while resisting the urge to push up. Let yourself be lifted with as little effort as possible. It's here you can imagine bringing the front of the heart toward the light of the sun, as if to allow the sun to ignite the light in your own heart. Imagine filling your heart with warmth, compassion, and love. Thus, we train ourselves to be softer and lighter, and trust the buoyancy of our own being.

Benefits: The cobra pose stretches and expands the chest and lungs, increases flexibility in the spine, improves blood flow to and from the heart, and opens and improves the flow of energy between the heart and arms. This pose can also help release tension in the back, shoulders, and neck. When done on the floor, it stimulates the stomach and digestion, and tones the abdominal muscles and reproductive organs.

Contraindications: If you have an abdominal aortic aneurysm, use the chair version so you are not lying on your belly. If you have mobility issues that interfere with moving up or down from the floor, you may also prefer the seated chair version.

The Practice of Cobra on the Floor

- Lie on the floor on your stomach.
- Feel the space in the back of your heart, and breathe as if your heart is breathing in and breathing out.
- Notice any feelings that arise.
- Begin to slide your legs together (they don't have to touch).
- Bend your elbows and plant your palms on the floor in line with your armpits.
- Rest your forehead on the floor.
- Brush the forehead, nose, and chin against the floor as you raise your head and follow the lift into the heart.

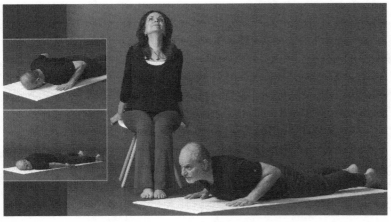

Figure 2.6. Cobra.

- Hold the pose effortlessly as you breathe.
- When you feel ready, slowly lower down on an exhale, brushing the chin and nose, and then placing the forehead on the floor.
- Practice 2 more times.
- When finished, turn your head to one side and rest. Let out a sigh through the mouth and relax completely. Be still and listen.

The Practice of Cobra in a Chair

- Sit comfortably in a chair.
- Hold the sides of the chair or let your hands rest in your lap.
- Lower your chin to your chest and round your spine.
- As you breathe naturally, start to lift your chin and lift your spine.
- Let your chest expand and your shoulders roll back gently (grab the chair to lift more).
- Keep the breath flowing, and hold the pose as long as it feels comfortable.
- Slowly lower the chin and round the spine.
- Now return to the center and relax. Listen.

When you do this pose every day, you will find new ways to connect to it and new things it can teach you about yourself. In time you may notice your shoulders freer, your back stronger, your heart lighter, and your awareness more embodied.

Half Locust
Nourishing and cleansing are both important aspects of health. Not only do we need to nourish ourselves, but cleansing is an

equally important aspect of health and healing. Eating a cleansing diet and doing practices that help us cleanse are important. We all know what it feels like when our house gets cluttered. We also know the feeling of spaciousness after taking those bags of clothes or unused items to a donation center. Our bodies need to be able to cleanse effectively or our energy starts to stagnate. We feel heavy and full. Toxins start to build up. Doing a fast or cleanse is one way, but making sure our elimination system is in good working order is another. Using the practice of half locust can be helpful in maintaining healthy elimination, as it supports the peristaltic action of the colon. Cholesterol is also stored in the colon, so healthy elimination encourages lower cholesterol levels.

Energetically, when we start to let go of the things we don't need anymore, we begin to create space. We stop carrying things we don't need both physically and emotionally. We clear the way for our own body to work more effectively and more efficiently.

Benefits: The half locust pose strengthens the low back, legs, and hips. It stimulates the endocrine and reproductive systems and improves peristalsis and elimination.

Contraindications: It's important to use the chair version if you have an abdominal aortic aneurysm or mobility issues that interfere with moving up or down from the floor. If you have chronic low back or neck pain, consider using the chair version.

The Practice of Half Locust on the Floor

- Lie on the floor on your stomach.

- Tuck your arms under you with your palms on your thighs (with hip bones on forearms). You can also let your arms rest alongside the body, if that's more comfortable.

- Start with your chin or forehead on the floor.

- Stretch out through your right leg and raise it slowly away from the floor. Keep breathing smoothly. Keep the leg extended as if reaching through the toes.

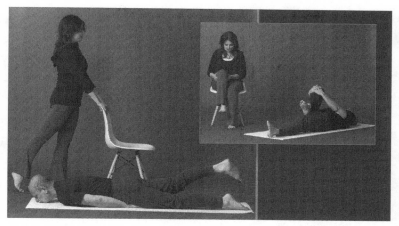

Figure 2.7. Half Locust.

- Slowly lower on an exhalation breath.
- Now practice on the opposite side.
- When you finish, turn the head to one side and let go.
- Sigh and relax. Imagine tension exiting through the soles of the feet.
- Now, gently roll to your back and draw one knee to the chest, then release it.
- Practice on the other side, releasing any held tension in your low back as you move.
- Rest and be still.

The Practice of Half Locust Using a Chair

- Stand using the back of a chair for support in front of you.
- Hold onto the chair with both hands.
- Step the right foot back while keeping the ball of the foot on the floor behind you.

Optional: You can also try to balance by lifting the foot a couple inches away from the floor.

- Hold this for a few breaths.
- Release by stepping the foot forward.
- Practice on the opposite side.
- Now sit in the chair.
- Lift under the right leg with both hands as you bring the foot off the floor and the knee/thigh closer to your torso as you gently lean forward.
- Lower slowly and practice on the opposite side.
- Practice a few times on each side alternating (this improves peristalsis).
- When finished, close your eyes, rest, and listen.

Seated Forward Bend

The practice of forward bending teaches us to let go of what is happening around us and turn inward. We begin to fold into our hearts and rest in our own inner wisdom. By following the flow of energy inward, we start to move into a quieter space. The external environment drifts away, and we meet ourselves in a deeper way. Here the nervous system can calm down, and there is an opportunity to let go of whatever we are holding, so we can settle even more.

Forward bends are not about *how far* you can go, but rather *how deeply* you can let go. Less is more, and when you give up the struggle and let the body unfold at its own pace you are learning about surrender. This practice helps us understand how to live in the natural flow of life by surrendering to what *is*. We give up the push and let ourselves be pulled by the deeper wisdom of our own bodies, trusting we will find our way.

Benefits: The forward bend pose improves flexibility of the spine, shoulders, hamstrings, and hips. It helps stretch the back and improves awareness of the backside of the body and heart. This pose also encourages "letting go" while calming the nervous system and the mind, promoting introspection.

Contraindications: If you have low back concerns, try using a folded pillow at your abdomen for support, and try doing less. For conditions such as glaucoma or a detached retina, you may consider keeping your chin lifted during practice.

The Practice of Seated Forward Bend on the Floor

- Sit on the floor with one pillow under the buttocks and another pillow under the backs of the knees.

- Place your hands on your thighs, and as you exhale, begin to slide forward. Allow your hands to slide down your legs.

- Keep the breath flowing as you bring your chin toward your chest, your abdomen toward your thighs, and your hands sliding toward your knees or shins.

- Rest when you find a comfortable edge; if you have gone too far, come back a little bit.

- Loosen your effort, relax your heart.

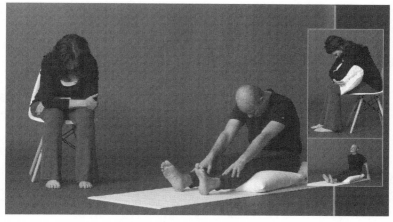

Figure 2.8. Seated Forward Bend.

- Breathe as if the back of your heart is breathing.
- After several breaths, slowly slide back up to center.
- Place your hands on the floor behind you for support as you gently press while you lengthen and lift the spine.
- Repeat 1 more time at your own pace.

The Practice of Seated Forward Bend in a Chair

- Sit comfortably in a chair.
- Place your hands on your thighs, and with an exhale breath begin to slide forward from the pelvis. Keep the breath flowing.
- Bring your chin toward your chest.
- Fold your forearms onto your thighs and rest there.
- Let your breath flow, and breathe as if the back of your heart is breathing.
- If you would like extra support, you can fold a pillow and place it against your abdomen and thighs.
- After several breaths, slowly press or slide back up the legs.
- Let your shoulders roll back and down, and relax.

Seated Spinal Twist

On a physical level, the practice of the seated spinal twist improves the overall flexibility of the spine. It encourages us to find a little bit of movement in a lot of places rather than a lot of movement in just a few places. This helps bring balance and awareness to areas in the spine that are moving too little or moving too much. As you twist, the organs begin to shift and move, creating some pressure and infusing them with fresh blood and energy. On an emotional level, the twist is asking us to "look around" and open our awareness to what is happening around us. It encourages us to take in another perspective and let it expand our view. So often we get stuck only seeing what is in front of us. We work for a goal, and the goal is always in the future. We begin to lose sight of anything else. The twist is asking us to be present and incorporate this broader view into our currently held ideas and beliefs. It begins to widen our view and prepare us to live in harmony with everything and everyone around us.

Benefits: The spinal twist pose improves flexibility of the spine, promotes blood flow to the internal organs, tones the nervous system, and broadens perspective.

Contraindications: If you have back, neck, hip, and knee issues, consider using the chair version.

The Practice of Seated Spinal Twist on the Floor

- Sit on the floor with your legs stretched out in front of you. Feel free to put a pillow under your buttocks to provide a lift for your spine.
- Bend your right knee and place your foot on the floor to the inside of your left calf or thigh.
- Hold onto your right knee with your left hand (simply grab your knee with the opposite hand).

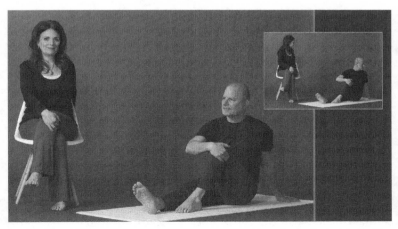

Figure 2.9. Seated Spinal Twist.

- Use your right hand placed on the floor behind you for support.
- Find a gentle lift in your spine as you begin to initiate a twist from the base of the spine up through the neck. Let the breath flow naturally.
- Let your eye gaze rest effortlessly to the space behind you.
- Take several breaths as you lengthen and soften.
- When you feel ready, slowly unwind back to center.
- Repeat on the opposite side. Relax and observe.

The Practice of Seated Spinal Twist in a Chair

- Sit in a chair with both feet on the floor.
- Cross your right leg over your left (you can leave both feet on the floor if crossing is uncomfortable).
- Place your left hand on your right knee.
- Place your right hand on the chair behind you for support.
- Find a gentle lift in your spine and begin to initiate a twist from the base of the spine up through the neck. Let the breath flow naturally.
- Let your eye gaze rest effortlessly to the space behind you.
- Take several breaths as you lengthen and soften.
- When you feel ready, slowly unwind back to center.
- Repeat on the opposite side.
- Relax and observe.

Modified Shoulder Stand

This posture is often called the pose of two waterfalls. Lying down with the legs placed on a chair gives a rest to the veins in the legs and allows the blood to flow with gravity back to the heart. With the pillows under the buttocks and the head, the blood is pooled first in the abdomen and low back, creating the first waterfall. The pillow under the buttocks lifts and carries blood to the neck, creating a second waterfall by bringing blood and energy to the carotid arteries. This sends the message to the brain that the heart has enough blood, and it doesn't need to pump as much. In turn, this lowers heart rate and blood pressure, resting the heart. This practice also brings blood, energy, and balance to the thyroid gland (the master gland that regulates hormone functions). It also drains the lymphatic system, which is not a pumped system. With the legs on the chair, it rests the muscles of the low back, relieving low back tension and tightness. This pose is quieting for the nervous system, mind, and heart. It is considered one of the most restorative poses for the heart and nervous system. It can be practiced for 1 minute and up to 10 minutes depending on your comfort levels.

When practicing in a chair, the benefits are slightly different since the legs are not resting above the heart. The chair version does, however, allow the legs to rest up off the floor, which supports the return of blood from the legs to the heart (also known as venous return). By dropping the chin slightly and resting, the nerves from the spinal cord to the brain send a message to the sympathetic nervous system (responsible for fight or flight) to power down. This upregulates the parasympathetic nervous system, which triggers the relaxation response.

Benefits: The modified shoulder stand lowers blood pressure and heart rate, drains the lymphatic system, relieves varicose and shattered veins, and brings blood flow and balance to the thyroid gland. It also helps alleviate low back discomfort, brings blood to the brain, and quiets the mind and the nervous system.

Variation: If there is any discomfort or pressure in the head when both legs are up on the chair, take one leg down and do the pose with only one leg on the chair at a time.

Contraindications: With any of the following conditions, the practice of modified shoulder stand should be done sitting in a chair: diabetes with retinopathy, detached retina, eye disease, history of stroke, menstruation, GERD (reflux), hiatal hernia, cervical/spinal arthritis, labile hypertension, carotid stenosis.

The Practice of Modified Shoulder Stand on the Floor

You will need one sturdy chair and two or three pillows for this posture.

- Lie on the floor and place two or three pillows close to your side.
- Place one leg on the seat of a chair. The legs will be supported from the back of the knee to the heel of the foot.
- Lift up and place one pillow under the buttocks and one or two pillows under the back of the head.
- Gently place the second leg up on the chair and relax.

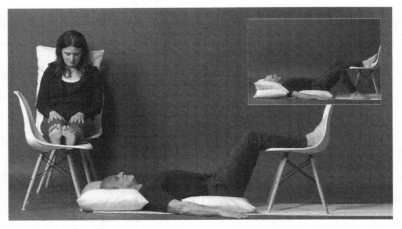

Figure 2.10. Modified Shoulder Stand.

- If there is too much pressure in the head, work with one leg up on the chair at a time.

- Relax; bring your attention to the heart and imagine your heart breathing.

The Practice of Modified Shoulder Stand in a Chair

You will need two sturdy chairs and two or three pillows for this posture.

- Place one chair up against a wall for support.
- Sit on that chair and use another chair for your legs.
- Place both legs up on the second chair.
- Place a pillow against the wall for your head to rest on.
- Let your chin soften toward your chest.
- Arms and hands can rest in your lap or down alongside the body.
- Take several breaths here, and breathe as if your heart is breathing. Relax.

Note: *You may consider using an imagery practice from chapter 6 while you rest here.*

The Practice of Fish

The practice of fish pose can begin to reverse some of the tension and tightness in the shoulders and chest that come from protecting the heart. The trauma of heart disease often leaves the heart feeling vulnerable and in need of the sheltering embrace of the shoulders. This can create a postural pattern that leaves the shoulders rounded and tense. It's not only heart disease that can cause this kind of pattern, but when our hearts feel vulnerable in general, we might protect our feelings and emotions in this same way. As we begin to explore the openness of this pose, we start to trust ourselves to hold those feelings with tenderness and compassion so we can embrace the new feelings of openness and vulnerability that arise.

Benefits: The fish pose improves flexibility of the spine, enhances blood flow to the heart and lungs, and promotes blood flow to the thyroid gland (the master gland and hormone regulator). It also opens the pathway between the heart and arms and improves posture, especially in the upper back and shoulders.

Contraindications: With any of the following conditions, the practice of fish can be done sitting in a chair: diabetes with retinopathy, cervical arthritis, carotid stenosis, history of stroke, eye diseases (glaucoma, detached retina, retinopathy), sternal wound when not fully healed, frequent dizziness.

Use of imagery: It can be fun to imagine yourself as a starfish sitting at the bottom of the ocean spread out in the sand as the water (breath) washes over you.

- While in the fish pose, begin to inhale from your heart to your feet and exhale from your feet back to your heart. Let the breath flow with ease as you seamlessly weave your breaths together, practicing for a few breaths.

- Now inhale from your heart to your fingers and exhale from your fingers to your heart, practicing again for a few breaths.

- Lastly inhale from your heart to the crown of your head and exhale from the crown to your heart, breathing smoothly and evenly.

- When you finish, let your breath land in your heart and breathe as if your heart is breathing.

The Practice of Fish on the Floor
You will need two or three pillows for this posture.

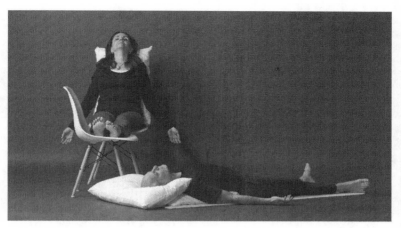

Figure 2.11. Fish.

- Sit on the floor with one pillow placed behind you length-wise to support the spine.

- Place a second pillow across the top edge of the first pillow.

- Support yourself as you lie over the pillows, allowing the bottom edge of the first pillow to rest at the base of the spine and the top edge of the second pillow to support you up to the middle of your ears.

- If needed, you can add another pillow under the backs of your knees to relax the low back.

- Allow the head to rest back, with the chin slightly lifted.

- Adjust the pillows for best support and comfort.

- Please note that if you have any of the listed contraindications you will need to adjust the second pillow so the head is not tilted back.

- Rest your arms comfortably away from the body, with palms up or down.

- Breathe as if your breath was opening a passageway from your heart to your fingers and your fingers to your heart.

Or you can use the suggested imagery and breathing of a starfish mentioned above.

- When finished, gently release by putting your hands under the back of your head and bringing your head to a neutral position. Bend the knees and roll onto one side.

The Practice of Fish in a Chair

You will need two sturdy chairs and two or three pillows for this posture.

- Place the back of one chair against a wall, so it's steady.
- Sit on that chair and place the legs up on the second chair.
- Place one pillow behind your back lengthwise along the spine from the base of the spine to the neck.
- Use a second pillow to support the neck and allow the head to rest back on the wall (this may take some adjusting, but you want support through the neck as the head extends back to rest on the wall).
- The chin is slightly lifted as the chest gently expands and the shoulders relax.
- Let the breath flow from the heart to the hands and the hands to the heart.
- Stay as long as it is comfortable and then gently release.

The practice of postures can be followed with a practice of relaxation and/or meditation from the chapters that follow. When these postures are done all together and in the order presented here, they can have a powerful effect on health and healing. With practice, patience, and commitment, these simple yet profound movements can begin to change the flow of energy in the body, rewire your nervous system, and change your mindset.

When we are living in our bodies with the sense of residency that postures provide, we become stewards of this precious body. We begin to move with an ease and grace that informs the way we live our lives. It's then that we can begin to listen to our own inner wisdom.

Relaxation

Creating Space and Letting Go

"The time to relax is when you don't have time for it."
—SYDNEY J. HARRIS[1]

A CENTERING MOMENT

Using Breath to Relax Areas of Tension in the Body

- Sit or lie down.

- Soften the gaze of your eyes.

- Take several conscious, slow, deep breaths.

- As you settle in, begin to turn your attention inward, as if to feel yourself from the inside.

- Notice any held tension in your body or mind. Just simply notice, no need to judge.

- Take a deep inhale, and as you exhale, begin to send a wave of relaxation over the body from top to toe. Repeat this several times, slowly.

- Imagine the breath smoothing out any tension that is within your reach, any tension you are willing and able to let go of.
- Pause for a moment and observe.
- Now send the breath directly into the specific areas of tension or tightness. Breathe as if you are breathing in, around, and through these areas. Allow the breath to unwind and dissolve any remaining tension within your reach.
- Now close your eyes and be still. Notice how you feel.

"Just relax." We hear this often when we're nervous, afraid, anxious, or excited. This phrase seems to be what friends and family offer as an antidote to our stress. The phrase itself sounds almost cavalier or trite. It sounds like it should be simple, but how do we do it and what does it mean? What seems relaxing for some may not be relaxing for others. I often hear people talk about their relaxing hobbies, like reading, golfing, knitting, or bird-watching. Other people turn to happy hour and prescription drugs to take the edge off.

While a few of those options may work in the short term, the effects are often fleeting. Some of these methods may be less harmful than others, yet none of them give us the internal skills to manage our stress. All these choices leave us reliant on something outside of us to fix a problem that is inside of us.

We want solutions that are lasting and helpful to manage our stress, but how do we truly rest our body and mind so we can do so? How do we experience deep relaxation? Relaxation is a learned and conscious letting go. Just like a computer needs to be rebooted regularly to run efficiently, so do we. The practice of relaxation is the reset button.

Relaxation is a way to power down the body and mind. Many people don't know what it feels like to be awake and relaxed. For example, they may experience just two states of consciousness, being awake and stressed or asleep and relaxed. When my sister was working a corporate job, she used to drive up to visit me and spend the weekend. It was a three-hour door-to-door drive. The minute she arrived, I would invite her to sit down and relax while I made some food. After a few minutes, she would be sound asleep. The stress of the week and the drive left her in deep need of relaxation, and sleep was the only way her body knew to reset and recover. Yet even sleep doesn't ensure relaxation. Often our sleep can be fitful, interrupted, and agitated, leaving us exhausted and depleted. When we *practice relaxation*, there's an opportunity to train our bodies and minds to be awake, alert, *and* deeply relaxed.

When we sleep, we are unconscious. In deep relaxation, we are super conscious, offering us the experience of being awake, alert, yet fully relaxed. Simply put, the difference between relaxation and sleep is *consciousness*. When we are relaxed and conscious, we can heal more effectively because this brings us back into balance, also known as homeostasis. It's in this place of balance that healing occurs naturally. Practicing daily relaxation has been one of the most powerful tools I have used to facilitate healing, with others and with myself.

Many cardiac patients I have worked with don't even realize how much tension they are holding until they practice deep relaxation. It often takes illness or in more extreme cases disease for some to wake up to these deeply held patterns. Often someone will come up to me after the practice with tears in their eyes and say, "I had no idea how tense and unsettled I was until I felt myself relax." We tend to live into our tensions and ignore them. We stop noticing that our shoulders are squeezed up next to our ears until we finally let them soften. These held tensions in the body can be connected to deeply held emotions such as anger, grief, or resentment. When we relax, we not only let go of the held physical pattern, but over time we find it easier to let go of and soften the underlying emotion that goes with it. When we practice regularly, it can be a way to stop the stockpile of held emotional tension in our bodies.

Sleep plays many roles in the maintenance of our mental and physical health. Sleep and sleep disorders are also implicated in the risk of heart disease and other disorders.[2] Deep, progressive relaxation has been shown to influence sleep as well as anxiety. In 2020 a study of COVID-19 patients showed that progressive muscle relaxation significantly reduced anxiety and improved sleep, resulting in faster healing.[3] The practice of progressive relaxation can play an important role in improving the overall quality and duration of sleep, and in some cases, it can rest the body and mind deeper than sleep.[4]

In many ancient traditions, they speak of not exhausting yourself before sleep but rather, to sleep when you still have energy from the day. This is so you can begin to store that energy for healing, rather than using up all your reserves each day. This kind of age-old wisdom is helpful when we look at the numbers of Americans who suffer from adrenal fatigue, a state that leaves us feeling exhausted and depleted even after we rest.[5] We just keep borrowing from our adrenal glands without giving back, without resting properly to heal. It's during sleep that the organs and glands are recharged and nourished. If we sleep when we are exhausted, we are using up all of our reserves and won't have the energy to repair and recharge ourselves. Deep relaxation provides the recovery our bodies and minds so deeply need.

Deep relaxation not only relaxes the body and supports better sleep, but there is evidence to show that it can lower blood pressure. Studies suggest that the practice of deep systematic relaxation, also known in the yoga tradition as savasana, is extremely beneficial in lowering blood pressure. In one study, researchers found that blood pressure could be controlled with regular relaxation techniques in 65 percent of patients. The researchers did not use any drug intervention to achieve this response and reported that if patients stopped practicing, their blood pressure rose significantly to pre-intervention levels.[6]

When I was working in the hospital teaching these techniques to heart patients, the nurses were so impressed with the changes they saw in our participants after the relaxation exercises that they decided to do a little experiment on their own. If a participant in our program came in with high blood pressure, they would record the numbers, and then they would take their blood pressure again right after the relaxation exercise. In every person, the numbers would change, often dramatically. This gave the participants hope and motivation to keep practicing each day. Over time, many of them were able to reduce their prescribed blood pressure medications. Over time, their bodies began to heal.

GETTING TO KNOW YOUR BODY
The Nervous System
When talking about the practice of relaxation, it is helpful to understand the role of the autonomic nervous system. This system controls involuntary actions, such as the beating of your heart and the widening or narrowing of your blood vessels. When something goes wrong in this system, it can cause serious problems, including blood pressure, heart, and breathing issues.

The autonomic nervous system is one of the major neural pathways activated by stress.

There are two branches of the autonomic nervous system that work together: the sympathetic and parasympathetic.

The sympathetic nervous system helps us respond in a crisis, initiating a series of changes in the body by activating the stress hormones known as norepinephrine, adrenaline, and cortisol. This in turn raises blood pressure and heart rate, sending more blood and oxygen to the large muscles, allowing us to fight or flee if we are in danger or responding to a crisis. This is often referred to as the "fight or flight" response.

When the sympathetic nervous system is chronically upregulated or activated, it increases the stress hormones in the bloodstream. This increases heart rate and constricts blood vessels, which then raises blood pressure so we can respond quickly to an incoming threat. These hormones can even cause your palms to sweat, your mouth to dry out, and your limbs to feel light, creating a heightened sense of awareness. When we don't allow this system to downregulate or rest, it keeps responding to every situation as if it were acute, and then the state of hyperarousal becomes chronic. When stress is chronic, it can lead to disease.[7]

In contrast, the parasympathetic nervous system helps us recover from stressful events. It lowers blood pressure and heart rate and is often what is called the "rest and digest" part of the nervous system. It has been coined the "relaxation response," which returns our system to a state of balance.

We must remember that it's not *just* the stressor itself, but our reaction to it that can cause this series of events within our nervous system. While someone might respond to a traffic jam by screaming at the cars in front of them, another person may take a few deep breaths and relish that moment of stillness, using that time to calm down and unwind from the business of the day. These different reactions will create different nervous system responses.

Unfortunately, in the first scenario, the cascade of stress hormones is almost immediate, and the effects of adrenaline can last up to an hour, even after you've been removed from the stressful situation.[8] The good news is, we have a choice in how we want to respond, even though it may not feel that way when we are in the midst of a difficult situation. Stress management gives us the tools to change the way we react and respond to stressors, in turn retraining the nervous system. Instead of feeling like our response is automatic and we have no control over it, we can see and feel the difference in the way we respond when we practice skills such as daily deep relaxation.

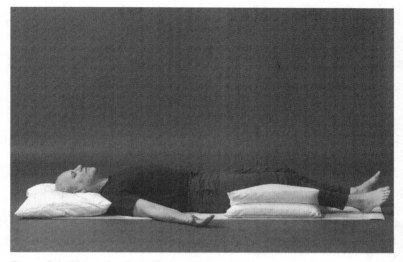

Figure 3.1. Relaxation Pose/Corpse Pose.

Yoga has long been touted as a powerful tool to manage stress and induce a sense of peace and well-being. Certain yoga practices can downregulate the sympathetic response and upregulate the parasympathetic response, or the "relaxation response." A study published in the *Journal of the Association of Physicians of India* found that yoga helped decrease sympathetic nervous system activity and dissipate the stress response that leads to high blood pressure. The authors concluded that yoga plays an important role in reducing the risk of mild to moderate hypertension.[9]

The practice of deep relaxation is most often done lying down in what the yoga tradition calls *savasana*, which translates to "corpse pose." While the position itself looks like a corpse, it's ultimately about letting go. To some, that sounds scary or uncomfortable, but that ability to let go can have a profound effect on your own health and well-being. Years ago, I went to a week-long seminar in Los Angeles where the Dalai Lama was teaching. I'll never forget one of his core teachings. He said, "Practice dying every day." This is how we learn to live more fully in the present moment and to overcome our fears of death and dying. For some of us, the fear of death is so strong that a practice like this can help unwind that fear so we can recognize the importance of our lives. Deep relaxation practiced in the corpse pose is a practice of learning to die, of letting go. It teaches us to let go of the future and release the past, so that we can live more fully and completely in this moment.

THE MAYA KOSHAS

When we practice relaxation, we're able to integrate ourselves on many levels, which allows us to heal and become more whole. These practices are meant to relax not only our physical body but also our subtle bodies, which cover our pure self or light within. In our Western culture, we see ourselves as having one body, but the yogis recognize five subtle bodies called the Maya Koshas. *Maya* means "illusion" and *Kosha* means "envelope" or "covering." Many of us, especially in the West, are trained to believe that we are our coverings, but this is an illusion. Beneath all these coverings is our true self, our light. That is really our true nature.

Ancient yogis understood these subtler bodies and the need to integrate them on a deep level for healing to occur. Author and teacher Nischala Joy Devi speaks of these sheaths during the practice of relaxation in her book *The Healing Path of Yoga*.[10] She talks about how we can observe them, integrate them, and ultimately transcend them to experience ourselves and our own inner light. This is done through the process of relaxing *from the outside in.*

The Food Body

During deep relaxation, we start by relaxing the outermost body. This is called the *Ana Maya Kosha*, which means "food body." The food body is what we know as our physical form. Our flesh, bones, muscles, organs, and glands are all included in this body. So when we are practicing relaxation, we start by allowing the muscles, bones, and even the organs to relax. This can be done

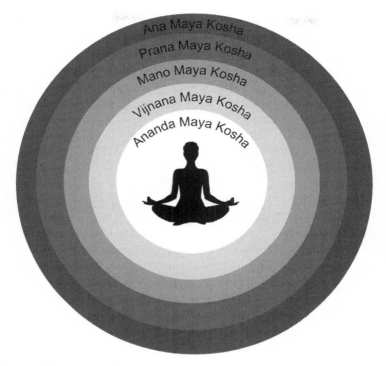

Figure 3.2. The Maya Koshas.

by squeezing and relaxing the muscles systematically, or it can be done by mentally traveling through the body and gently guiding each area to relax. Just relaxing physically can be very helpful, but as you experience the integration of the subtle bodies, this practice becomes deeply transformative.

The Energy Body
The next body is called the *Prana Maya Kosha*, which means "energy body" or "breath body." This is the body underneath our physical form that we refer to as our energy body. When we are with someone, we may not notice what they are wearing or how they look on the outside, but we may feel something from

them. We feel their energy. We may even say, "Wow, that person had really nice energy." This is the Prana Maya Kosha we are experiencing.

After relaxing our physical body, we begin to breathe as if the whole body is breathing. We may even imagine taking the breath into any areas of lingering tension to breathe and soften them even more. This helps us connect with our energy body. We may start to feel a bit transparent as we loosen the edges and boundaries of the body. We may even notice a sense of freedom from our physical form, as physical pain and discomfort begin to ease or disappear. Here we can experience ourselves connected to the energy of every living, breathing being. We begin to feel less alone, and more like we are part of something much larger than ourselves.

The Mind Body

Next, we become aware of the everyday mind and the senses. This subtle body is called the *Mano Maya Kosha*, which means "mind body." This is where our thoughts, feelings, and sensations reside. It's where we store our emotional pain, as well as all the impressions from the senses. Once we have slowed down the physical body and observed the breath body, we can begin to notice our everyday thoughts and feelings as they arise. As thoughts and feelings come into our awareness, we continue to use our breath to relax any lingering thoughts or feelings.

Wisdom Body

As the body, breath, and mind begin to rest in alignment, a deeper sense of stillness and peace will emerge. We become aware of the *Vijnana Maya Kosha*, which means "wisdom body." As we become aware of our own inner wisdom, we connect with our intuition and start to gain some perspective. To experience this subtle body, we begin to step back from the mind and emotions and bear witness to them. We observe without judging. We simply allow thoughts and feelings to arise, and we watch as they dissipate. We may even see the origin of thoughts and feelings. This observation gives rise to a deep sense of insight. We gently allow the mind to unwind as we hold a space that is free from all labeling, analyzing, ruminating, and judging.

At some point, the mind grows weary of witnessing thought and there is a pull to move deeper. Now we can begin the journey into that place of peace that lives deep within. We find ourselves resting deeply in a sense of stillness and joy. We may even sense that we are peace, we are joy, we are love.

The Bliss Body

Last, but certainly not least, we begin to access the *Ananda Maya Kosha*, which means "bliss body." It is here, in this blissful body, that we can experience the reflection of our own light and our own true self. As we rest here, we are connected to our own inner light, our own inner healer. And then we rest, in our own true nature.

After resting here, it is important to come out the same way we went in, so as not to disturb this deep sense of peace and integration. We begin to observe the mind, thoughts, and emotions as we take some slow, deep breaths, awakening the organs and then the extremities. It helps to allow the breath to redefine the edges and boundaries of the body and feel yourself fully present in the spaces of the body. Slowly move your fingers and toes as you transition back into the physical world around you, allowing yourself to integrate this feeling of peace into your life.

This process of relaxing through the different bodies takes us into the deepest parts of our being and allows us to relax and integrate each one of our five bodies. When we practice regularly, our whole being begins to shine from the *inside out*. We find ourselves moving through the day with more energy, grace, and even kindness. The things that used to bother us just don't seem to bother us in the same way. Our tolerance grows and our fuse gets longer.

We are more likely to respond to stressful situations with a sense of ease, and recover our sense of calm more quickly.

Practicing Relaxation

It may be helpful to record your own voice reading the practice so you can play it for yourself whenever you need it (or visit www .yourcenteredheart.com for guided audio practices). If you're reading these relaxation exercises into a recording device, remember to read slowly and softly and pause between sentences. It may be helpful to imagine you are reading with the intention to soothe a young child or someone you love.

See if you can set aside some of the concerns or worries you have. It can be helpful to imagine setting them aside in a basket, knowing you can pick them up later, if you want. I like to imagine them floating down the river. Here are a few other things to consider before practicing:

- Choose a time to practice when you will not be disturbed. Midday, late afternoon, before dinner, and before bed are just a few times that could work well.

- These relaxation practices can be done in any comfortable position. I recommend lying on your back if it's comfortable. If lying on your back is not comfortable, try lying on your side or stomach, or sitting in a chair.

- Use a pillow under your head and under the backs of your legs for comfort.

- Cover up with a blanket, since the practice of deep relaxation lowers blood pressure and heart rate, which can lower body temperature.

- Try to stay awake during this practice, but if you fall asleep, know that sleep is what you need. If you fall asleep every time you practice, you may want to explore getting more sleep or try sitting up to practice. Ideally, you are training yourself to be *awake and deeply relaxed* at the same time.

- Know that the effects are cumulative, so a daily practice is recommended.
- When you finish with your practice, transition slowly and take the calm, relaxed feeling with you into your life.

Remember that the peace and calm you feel after practicing is always there inside of you. It can't be gotten from the external world—not from acquiring possessions, positions, or even people. It only needs to be uncovered and remembered. These practices help you uncover and reclaim the calm within.

The Practice of Centering Relaxation
Lie down or sit in a chair and cover up. Use any props, pillows, or blankets to get comfortable.

- Begin with several conscious, slow, deep breaths.
- Let the breaths mark a transition from busyness to stillness, a transition from thinking and doing to feeling and being.
- Now notice the space around you and the space the body occupies on the floor.
- Allow the body to settle into that space each time you exhale.
- Begin to draw your attention inward and close your eyes.
- Let go of the mind's desire to travel outward with the senses.
- Be content to hold your attention inward now.
- Start to feel yourself from the inside.

- Take your awareness through the body and take notice of any tension you may be holding in the different parts of your body.
- Use your awareness and your gentle breath to begin to relax and unwind patterns of tension within your reach.
- Take your awareness to each of the areas where you are holding tension and begin to breathe in, around, and through these areas systematically. Gently encourage held tension to soften, dissolve, and dissipate.
- Now let yourself settle with any tension that remains. Settle with yourself, just as you are, without the push or pull of wanting things to be different. Be content to rest with all the current conditions and circumstances.
- Begin to allow your awareness to occupy all the spaces of your body.
- Breathe as if your whole body were breathing, as if the pores in your skin could breathe.
- The inhale breath brings in vitality and energy. It's nourishing.
- The exhale breath gets rid of toxins and anything you don't need anymore. It's cleansing.
- Feel the whole body breathing. Observe the wavelike motion of breath in the body (observe for 2 minutes).
- Now begin to narrow your awareness of breath. Draw your attention to the tip of your nose.
- Notice if one nostril is more open than the other. Just notice, no need to try to change anything. Begin to follow the breath as it passes from the tip of the nose to the center of the mind, and from the center of the mind to the tip of the nose.
- Trace and track the breath as it comes in and as it goes out.

- Let the breath rest in the foreground of your awareness.

- Let thoughts, feelings, and sensations settle into the background, like the snow in a snow globe settling to the bottom. The picture becomes clearer, more focused, still and calm.

- If you find thoughts finding their way back into your awareness, just pause and notice.

- Let go of analyzing, ruminating, or getting caught in the drama. Simply shift back to breath.

- Center yourself with each breath (practice centering for 3–5 minutes).

- When you feel ready to come out, let your breath spread out into the spaces of your body.

- Deepen the in breath and lengthen the out breath.

- Begin to breathe movement into the fingers and toes.

- Cup your hands and bring them over your eyes. Open your eyes into the cupped hands.

- Gently massage the facial muscles and the scalp with your fingertips.

- Slowly begin to move your body, rolling onto one side, and come back to a seated position.

- Take a few more conscious, slow, deep breaths and try to maintain this feeling of calm and centeredness as you go about your day/life.

The Practice of Systematic Deep Relaxation
Lie down or sit in a chair and cover up. Use any props, pillows, or blankets to get comfortable.

- Start to make a transition from all the duties and responsibilities of the day.

- Begin to notice how you feel.
- Allow the body to rest deeply and completely while the mind remains alert, awake, and fully relaxed.
- Gently send your awareness down the body to the soles of the feet.
- Now slowly direct relaxation to the soles of the feet and the toes, then to the tops of the feet and ankles. Relax.
- Send relaxation to the lower legs, knees, upper legs, and hip joints. Relax.
- Take several breaths as you relax the feet and legs.
- Find your awareness in the fingertips. Relax the fingers and hands, the wrists and the lower arms, the elbows and upper arms and shoulder joints.
- Take several breaths and completely relax the hands and arms.
- Now direct your awareness and send relaxation to the pelvic floor and buttocks.
- Relax the abdomen and the organs of the abdomen. Let go of any gripping or tension in the abdominal organs.
- Now bring your awareness to the area of the stomach and navel. Relax the stomach and the organs of digestion and assimilation.
- Relax the chest, ribs, and muscles between the ribs. Notice the ribs expand on the inhale, then notice the ribs contract on the exhale.
- Relax the diaphragm, the lungs, and even the bronchioles.
- Now relax the heart.
- Relax the physical heart, and relax the emotional heart as well. Soften. Let go.
- Soften the throat and the pit of the throat.

- Gently return your attention to the lower back.

- Relax the lower back and middle back. Rest the upper back and shoulder blades and the space between the shoulder blades.

- Imagine sending relaxation up through the center of the spine.

- Relax the back of the neck and the base of the skull, the hinges of the jaw, the chin, and the lips.

- Soften the mouth and the corners of the mouth, the gums and nerves of the teeth. Relax.

- Now rest the tongue and the roof of the mouth. Relax the nasal passages, sinuses, and nostrils.

- Notice the breath as it passes through the nostrils.

- Relax the cheeks and the eyes. Allow the eyes to soften in the sockets.

- Relax the eyebrows and the space between the eyebrows, the forehead, temples, ears, and scalp.

- Now relax the mind and any thoughts that linger in the mind.

- Begin to gather up any remaining tension from the body, any remaining tension from the mind, and send them out through the top of the head.

- Let go of any cares or worries, any fears or concerns.

- Relax completely and deeply from top to toe and toe to top (take a long, silent pause here).

- Notice the breath and how the body organizes around the natural rhythms of breath.

- Notice the mind and the thoughts that linger in the mind.

- Observe thoughts arising and dissipating.

- Bear witness to the mind without labeling or judging, without analyzing or ruminating.
- Now begin to move deeper as you search for that place of peace and stillness deep within.
- Allow yourself to rest in that center of stillness. Rest in your own true nature, deeply letting go (pause here for at least 2–5 minutes).
- From that place of stillness and peace, begin to observe the mind.
- Now notice the breath.
- As you deepen the in breath and lengthen the out breath, allow the breath to fill the spaces of the body.
- When you feel ready, begin to make a transition.
- Allow the breath to inspire some movement in the fingers and toes, in the ankles and wrists.
- Cup the hands and bring them over the eyes, then open the eyes into the cupped hands.
- Use the pads of the fingers to massage the forehead and scalp.
- When ready, stretch the body by reaching the arms over-head and pressing down through the soles of the feet.
- Bend the knees, roll to one side, and pause there.
- Make a slow transition back to sitting.
- Try to maintain this feeling of peace and calm as you go about your day/life.

The Practice of Tense and Relax

This is a long version of relaxation. Allow 20–25 minutes for this practice.

This practice is great when you haven't practiced any gentle movement before relaxing. Squeezing and tensing the muscles helps activate the body and takes the relaxation deeper.

- Lie on the floor in a comfortable position. Use pillows to prop for comfort and a blanket to cover up.
- Take a few slow, conscious, deep breaths as you begin to transition from all the duties and responsibilities of the day.
- Inhale and gently squeeze the right leg from the toes to the hip. Exhale with an audible sigh as you relax.
- Gently squeeze the left leg from the toes to the hip as you inhale. Exhale with an audible sigh as you relax.
- Inhale and gently squeeze the right arm from the fingers to the shoulder joint. Exhale with a sigh as you relax.
- Gently squeeze the left arm from the fingers to the shoulder joint as you inhale. Exhale with a sigh as you relax.
- Inhale, squeeze the buttocks. Exhale, relax.
- Inhale, expand the abdomen. Then let the abdomen completely relax as you exhale with an audible sigh.
- Now repeat the same sequence with the upper chest. Inhale, expand the upper chest, and relax as you exhale with an audible sigh.
- Leaving your arms relaxed on the floor, inhale and bring the shoulders up toward the ears. Exhale, relax.
- Inhale, bring the shoulders together in front of the chest. Exhale, relax.
- Inhale, press the shoulders away from the ears. Exhale, relax.
- Slowly lift the head up and then slowly lower it as you relax and sigh. (If you have neck pain, don't lift the head;

instead, roll the head from side to side and allow the neck to relax.)

- Inhale and gently squeeze together all the facial muscles, including the jaw, mouth, eyes, and forehead. Make a prune face. Exhale, relax.
- Let go completely (take a long pause here).
- Allow yourself to shift from thinking and doing to feeling and being.
- Now take the mind through the body, allowing each part of the body to relax even deeper.
- Mentally relax the feet, legs, and hips.
- Relax the hands, arms, and shoulders.
- Relax and soften the buttocks, abdomen, and chest.
- Soften the heart and the throat.
- Now send relaxation up through the center of the spine, and allow the muscles to loosen their hold around the bones. Observe as the back softens and broadens.
- Soften the neck, the muscles of the face, and the organs of sense (the mouth, nose, eyes, ears, and brain). Relax.
- Relax the temples, forehead, scalp, and top of the head.
- Completely relax the whole body.
- Now bring awareness to the breath; without trying to change the pattern, just observe the gentle flow of air as it comes in and as it goes out.
- Notice whatever thoughts or feelings come up, and allow them to arise and dissipate without labeling, analyzing, or ruminating.
- Begin to move deeper as you search for that place of peace and stillness deep within.
- Allow yourself to rest (pause here for 1–2 minutes).

- Notice as you begin to lose the edges and boundaries of the body for a more spacious version of yourself—as if to feel yourself connected to everything living and breathing. A sense of oneness.

- From this place of oneness, there is no separation between self and other, just a feeling of unity. You may even sense that you are peace, that you are awareness.

- Allow yourself to rest for 3–5 minutes.

- From that place of expansiveness and peace, begin to allow your awareness to rise to the surface.

- Notice the mind.

- Observe the breath.

- Allow the breath to become a little deeper.

Note: *You can end this practice here by moving fingers and toes and rolling to one side before sitting back up, or you can continue with a healing imagery practice.*

Healing Imagery Practice

- Imagine healing light or healing energy sitting above the crown of the head.

- Allow it to get brighter and stronger as you draw it into the body.

- Send it over the mind and down the spine, and through to the vital organs.

- Direct it down the arms to the fingers and down the legs to the toes.

- Let it touch every fiber of your being, every cell filling with this healing light or energy.

- Allow this healing light to create a powerful healing shift.

- Rest here for 1 minute.

- Slowly begin to move the fingers, toes, hands, and feet.
- Gently roll the arms and legs back and forth.
- When you are ready, slowly roll over onto the side, bend the knees, and come to a seated position.
- Make a gentle transition to movement when ready.

These practices of relaxation can have a deep and profound effect on the body, nervous system, mind, and heart. With time and practice you will begin to see the effects of these practices flowering in your life. There is a spaciousness that arises when we aren't trying to fill every second. When we know how to slow down and create space, the important things in life will present themselves without us having to chase them. With calm awareness, the world becomes clearer, and we are able to make more intentional choices. Sometimes the people around us will be the first to notice when we aren't practicing, and they are not shy about reminding us: "Hey, I think you might need to do your relaxation practice, I can tell you're not yourself." Once people see the changes in us, they want to support us in whatever is making us happy.

When I was teaching these techniques in a hospital program, one of the participants, a high-powered lawyer, came into class and exclaimed in his gruff manner, "I think something might be wrong with me." When I asked him to explain, he said, "Before when I was at work, I would walk out to the hallway to get coffee and everyone would scatter, like cockroaches. They actually feared me. Now when I come out of my office, people stand around and talk to me. They seem to *like me*. Isn't that weird?" When I asked him why that was a problem, he said, "Well, I'm not used to having friends and I'm not sure what to do with that." I looked at him and gently asked, "Could you enjoy it?" He smiled and my heart melted.

Tenderness and connection aren't a sign of weakness, but rather a testament to our personal power. Being relaxed and calm doesn't mean we lose our creative edge, our spunk, or even our sense of humor, it just allows us to manage our energy and choose how we want to use it.

We all know too well how it feels when we are unglued, dysregulated, and surly. It's not like we get up intending to be as awful as we can be that day. Being relaxed, by actually *practicing* deep relaxation, gifts us the opportunity to be our best selves. So the next time someone tells you to "just relax," know that it's not a command, but an invitation. An invitation to practice cultivating relaxation and peace from within. An invitation to find your centered heart.

CHAPTER 4

Breathing

Energy and Life Force

""The yogi's life is not measured by his days, but by the number of his breaths."

—B. K. S. IYNEGAR[1]

A CENTERING MOMENT

2-to-1 Breathing

- Sit comfortably (this can also be done standing).
- Soften the gaze of your eyes; feel free to close your eyes if you are sitting.
- As you settle in, begin to turn your attention to the breath passing through the nostrils.
- Without changing the breath, notice the length of the inhale and the length of the exhale.
- Gently observe the pattern.

- Now see if you can make the breaths even. For example, if you are inhaling to the count of 3, then try exhaling to the count of 3. This may take several breaths before you can find an easy, even breath rhythm.
- Allow this even breath rhythm to flow for several breaths.
- Now begin to allow the exhale to get longer. Over time, allow the exhale to be twice as long as the inhale. This may take several more breaths.
- Let this 2-to-1 pattern of breath continue to ebb and flow for a few moments.
- Notice how you feel. Let your breath return to a rhythm that feels right for you.

BREATHING IS CENTRAL TO LIFE. IT'S THE FIRST THING WE DO AS we enter this life, and it is the last thing we do as we exit. Breathing is one way we gather the energy we need to sustain the body and its activities; the other is through food. Think of how attentive most of us are to our diets, but rarely do we think of breathing in the same way. We can go almost three months without eating if we have water, but only 4 to 6 minutes without a breath. Our breath is *that* important. Other compelling breath facts reveal that:

- Seventy percent of the body's waste is carried out with the exhalation breath in the form of carbon dioxide. This is more than is carried out through the skin with perspiration, and more than the bladder or bowel with evacuation.[2]
- The average person breathes in the equivalent of 13 pints of air every minute and takes 20,000 breaths per day.[2]

- When resting, the average adult breathes around 12 to 20 times per minute.[3]
- Breathing is a system that is both automatic (autonomous nervous system) and under our conscious control.[4]

The importance of breath can't be underestimated. In the tradition of yoga, breath is what carries prana, or energy. Therefore, great importance is placed on the quality of our breathing, just like the importance of the quality of the food we eat. Additionally, the breath actually connects us to everything living and breathing. In nature, the plants and trees literally breathe in what we breathe out. And remarkably, we breathe in what the plants and trees breathe out. Simply put, we all breathe the same air. We are intimately connected to nature through our interdependence. Our relationship to nature through breath is a constant reminder of our oneness. The more attention we pay to breath, the more we strengthen our connection to all life. During a time when life feels so divisive, breath reaffirms our connection to each other and to the planet.

We are all breathing all the time, but for many of us, when we are under chronic stress our breath can become short and shallow. Often, I hear yoga teachers and breathing enthusiasts proclaim that there is a right or wrong way to breathe. I just want to say, if you're breathing, it's right. What is more true is that how we breathe can affect how we think and feel, and how we think and feel can affect how we breathe. Our breath patterns have consequences. My teacher, a swami, used to say that every disease has a breath pattern that precedes it. This would suggest that our breath patterns are integral to our physical health and well-being.

There have been studies conducted to investigate the use of simple breathing techniques on heart health. Research has shown that just 5 minutes of slow, deep, yogic breathing significantly decreases heart rate and systolic blood pressure in hypertensive patients.[5] It has been demonstrated that practices that include slowing the breath rate to about four breaths per minute, unlike our usual twelve to twenty breaths per minute, naturally calms the heart and may beneficially affect cardiovascular autonomic regulation in various cardiovascular diseases.[6] I have witnessed these kinds of results time and time again using slow, deep, yogic breathing in my own work with cardiac rehab patients. In addition, after seeing the results of this kind of intervention, many of the cardiac nurses started teaching these breathing practices to their other cardiac rehab patients.

Our breath is the link between the body and the mind. What happens in the mind gets reflected in the breath, and what happens in the breath gets reflected in the mind. For example, during a panic attack, the mind races and the breath becomes short and shallow. Short, shallow breathing can trigger the sympathetic nervous system and the fight or flight response. This releases adrenaline, a hormone that temporarily causes your breathing and heart rate to speed up and your blood pressure to rise. Yet if you pause and soften the pattern of breath, the mind begins to settle, and the panic shifts. By the same token, when the panic shifts, so does the breath rhythm.

Learning to adjust the breath rhythms can play an integral role in slowing the heart rate, resting the heart, and improving heart health and mental health. Many people experience shallow breathing and patterns of breath retention that are unconscious, caused by trauma, stress, or simply underutilization of full-breath patterns. For example, when we sit at a desk working all day, the breath may become shallow because we aren't moving, and we don't need a lot of oxygen to sit still. Yet if we do that day after day, we may start to lose the ability to breathe more deeply. Simple breath awareness techniques can call attention to these patterns and allow you to reshape the breath rhythms that aren't serving you. Breath awareness is a practice of getting curious about your own breath habits. Start by asking yourself these questions throughout the day: What is happening right now in my own breathing? Is it long or short? Is it deep or shallow? Shaky or at ease? Am I holding my breath? If so, when in my breath cycle am I holding?

You may find that just noticing your breath can be challenging; once you turn your attention to breath, you will immediately try to change it. Yet with practice, you will begin to observe your own patterns. From that place of awareness, we can begin to use breathing exercises, such as practicing slow, deep, yogic breathing, to help reset and retrain these habits. The exercises support the expansion and direction of breath and, more than anything, can provide us with more options for breath. This creates adaptability; in turn, being able to adapt affects our survival and our long-term health.

When we talk about slow, deep breathing and its effect on our health, it's important to understand the role of the diaphragm muscle. We often hear singers speak about using the support of the diaphragm when they are singing, but what is the role of this muscle in our breathing?

THE DIAPHRAGM MUSCLE

The diaphragm muscle, also known as the central tendon, is the muscle just above the stomach and just below the rib cage, separating the chest cavity from the abdomen. It's a dome-shaped muscle attached to your sternum (a bone in the middle of your chest), the bottom of your rib cage, and your spine. It flattens and spreads out on the inhale, and it contracts and moves up on the exhale. During the inhalation, the diaphragm muscle pulls air down into the gravity-dependent part of the lungs, acting much like a vacuum. This in turn causes the abdomen to expand. When we exhale, the diaphragm moves back up and presses the air out of the lungs, and the abdomen contracts.

The yogis recognized the importance of strengthening the diaphragm, since the degree to which we can get a deep breath depends in large part on the strength of the diaphragm muscle. Some say this is the most important muscle in the whole body, because without it we cannot breathe on our own.

One very simple way to begin to work with this muscle is to lie on your belly with your arms folded in front of you in what is called crocodile pose (see chapter 2 for a full description). Let your forehead rest on your forearms, allowing your upper chest to be up off the floor to send more weight to the diaphragm muscle. Let your legs rest a comfortable distance apart. You can experiment with a position that works for your body. As you focus on slow, long, deep breathing, the floor (the harder, the better) creates resistance for and puts pressure on the diaphragm. You may find that it takes a little work to breathe deeply. This simple practice not only allows you to locate and bring awareness to the diaphragm muscle, but also contributes to strengthening the muscle. Try it for 2 to 5 minutes.

Once you have located your diaphragm muscle, you're ready to begin your exploration into the breathing practices.

THE BREATHING PRACTICES

- Even Breathing
- 2-to-1 Breathing
- Abdominal Breathing
- Long, Wide, and Deep Breathing
- Three-Part Breathing
- Alternate Nostril Breathing
- Humming Breath

Notes for Breathing Practices:

- Try to practice in a well-ventilated room, or in fresh air.
- Start by just getting curious about your own patterns of breath. This is called breath awareness. It's done by checking in with your breathing and noticing the qualities of your breath throughout the day.

- When adopting a new breath rhythm, be gentle. Don't overbreathe or try too hard.

- Allow yourself to relax into the practice as much as possible.

- If you feel lightheaded or dizzy, stop and let your breath rhythm return to normal.

- Choose one practice and work with it for a few days or even weeks before adding other practices.

- Eventually some of the practices can be done together.

- If you have difficulty breathing such as COPD or asthma, it's best not to overfocus on breath. Rather begin with the practice of relaxation (found in chapter 3) and in time, gently begin to guide the breath rhythms.

Even Breathing

Research has shown that slow, deep, *even* breathing can lower blood pressure and heart rate in just 5 minutes.[7] This claim may seem almost miraculous to those who have never experienced the effects of slow, deep breathing, but it is not news to those who practice yoga. It has long been understood how quickly breathing can affect not only heart rate and blood pressure, but the nervous system and the mind. Even breathing sets a foundation for all the other practices of breathing. The great part is that you can adapt this practice to use anywhere at any time. The breath is always with you, and you have the ability to control the rhythm with just your attention.

The Practice of Even Breathing

- Begin lying down or sitting up.
- Gently close your eyes and relax the body.
- Turn your attention to the breath.

- After a few relaxed breaths, begin to keep count of the length of your inhale breath.

- Once you find a natural, relaxed inhale count, begin to let the exhale count match the inhale count. If your inhale count is 4, let your exhale count be 4 as well. This may take several breaths, so be patient and don't force it.

- Continue this for 3–5 minutes.

- When finished, relax your effort, and let the breath return to a rhythm that is natural.

2-to-1 Breathing

2-to-1 breathing is done by allowing the exhale breath to extend twice as long as the inhale breath. This is done by observing the natural rhythm and flow of the inhale and then counting each inhalation breath. Once you find a comfortable count, allow the out breath to extend twice as long. This may take several breaths before the rhythm takes hold. You might start with an inbreath of 3 to 4 counts and slowly extend the exhale to 6 or 8. Don't force it. Just let it take shape over several breaths.

It would seem that if slow, even breathing could lower heart rate and blood pressure, then 2-to-1 breathing should have a similar effect. Indeed it does. Again research has found that just 5 to 7 minutes daily of 2-to-1 breathing comprehensively affected the autonomic nervous system, and as a result helped in the management of hypertension or high blood pressure.[8]

You may notice that with just a few minutes of practice, a calm feeling arises. I often use this practice when I am feeling over my edge. It signals the parasympathetic nervous system and upregulates a relaxation response.

The Practice of 2-to-1 Breathing

- Begin lying down or sitting up.

- Gently close your eyes and relax the body.

- Turn your attention to the breath.

- After a few relaxed breaths, begin to keep count of the length of your inhale breath.

- Once you find a natural, relaxed inhale count, begin to let the exhale count extend twice as long as the inhale count. If your inhale count is 4, let your exhale count lengthen to 8. This may take several breaths, so be patient and don't force it.

- Continue this for 3–5 minutes.

- When finished, relax your effort, and let the breath return to a rhythm that is natural.

Abdominal Breathing (Long Breathing)

As mentioned above, during the inhalation, the diaphragm muscle pulls air down into the gravity-dependent part of the lungs. This in turn causes the abdomen to expand. When we exhale, the diaphragm muscle moves back up and presses the air out of the lungs, and the abdomen contracts. With stress or trauma, this movement can get confused and cause what is called "paradoxical breathing." This is where the stomach and abdomen move in on the inhale and out on the exhale—the opposite of abdominal breathing. Over time this can cause the breath to become more and more shallow. This shallow breathing upregulates the sympathetic nervous system and signals the adrenals to produce more adrenaline. The adrenaline creates a rapid heartbeat, anxiety, and more shallow breathing, and the cycle goes on and on. It can be a hard cycle to break. By bringing attention to the diaphragm and abdomen, a new habit can be created and the natural breath rhythm restored.

In the book *Conscious Breathing* by Gay Hendricks, PhD, the connection of paradoxical breathing and heart disease is brought to light in research with 153 cardiac patients in a Minneapolis cardiac unit. All had suffered heart attacks, and every one of them was found to be a chest breather. Not a single one was using abdominal breathing. This finding is telling, and clearly points to the importance of not only breathing patterns that support heart health but the patterns that can contribute to the disease process as well.[9]

The Practice of Abdominal Breathing

- Begin by sitting in a chair or on the floor.
- Place one hand over your abdomen below the navel.
- Close your eyes and let your awareness connect to the breath.
- As you inhale, begin to exaggerate the expansion of the abdomen, as if to imagine blowing a balloon up in the abdomen.
- As you exhale, exaggerate the contraction of the abdomen as if the balloon were deflating.
- After exaggerating the movement, now relax your effort and let it become more natural.
- Practice for several minutes and then release the hand and open the eyes.

Long, Wide, and Deep Breathing

As we continue to explore the breath, it's helpful to recognize that the breath has three directions or pathways it can take: long, wide, and deep.

With *long breathing*, the breath moves up and down. We can create this pattern by imagining the breath moving from the top of the head to the tips of the toes, and from the tips of the toes to the top of the head. To get familiar with this direction of breath, it can help to exaggerate the movement. Allow your breath to travel up and down the body slowly and smoothly. This encourages breath to move deep into the gravity-dependent part of the lungs. The force of the diaphragm moving down to let more air in causes the abdomen to rise as you inhale and to fall as you exhale. This is also referred to as abdominal breathing, as discussed above.

Note: Notice if the breath moves up to the crown of the head when you exhale or when you inhale. There isn't a right way to breathe, but it is interesting to notice your patterns. Can you change it? If you were breathing up on the inhale and down on the exhale, can you now try breathing up on the exhale and down on the inhale? Is one direction easier or more comfortable than the other?

With *wide breathing*, the rib cage is the focus. The breath moves from the center of the chest out to the side ribs, and from the side ribs to the center of the chest. To experience the pattern, imagine the breath gently pressing the ribs out to walls on either side of you as you inhale, and then imagine the breath moving back to the center of the chest as you exhale. The rib cage expands and contracts with this movement. Some people might call wide breathing diaphragmatic breathing since the focus is around the diaphragm region, but it's important to recognize that all breathing is diaphragmatic, so this term can be confusing.

Note: Another experiment would be to exhale and imagine the rib cage expanding out to either side, then inhale and imagine the breath returning to the heart—essentially the opposite of the above-mentioned pattern. If either of these patterns of breath feels unfamiliar, you may want to explore them from time to time as a way to become more familiar with different patterns of breath as a way to create more options and adaptability for breath.

With *deep breathing*, the upper lungs and upper chest are now brought into awareness. To experience this pattern, while sitting up, imagine that as you inhale the breath moves from your chest out to the wall in front of you, and as you exhale it returns and moves to the wall behind you. This requires the engagement of the upper chest muscles. If you do this practice while lying down, imagine that with the inhale the chest rises toward the ceiling; as you exhale, imagine the breath descending deep into the floor beneath you.

Note: Again, as an experiment, you might try to breathe the opposite way. While sitting in a chair, as you inhale the breath travels from the upper chest and reaches to the wall behind you, and as you exhale the chest moves to the wall in front of you. You can do this lying on the floor as well.

All three of these movements of breath are accessible to us throughout the day. With stress and trauma, we may get stuck in a pattern where we have limited access to one or more of these options. As we start practicing each of the exercises, our breathing becomes more flexible and adaptable, and we begin to gain access to all the directions of breath. In time, our connection to breath and our breathing capacity expands, and we gain access to the profound impact and power of the breath.

When we take a slow, deep breath and encourage the use of all three directions, this is called the three-part breath. It's helpful to work with each of these pathways separately before weaving them together.

Three-Part Breathing (Long, Wide, and Deep)

Three-part breathing refers to deep breathing that expands and contracts the abdomen, rib cage, and chest as you breathe. This type of breathing increases the capacity of the lungs, allowing us to take in about seven times the amount of oxygen as with a normal breath. Not only that, but three-part breathing helps reset the breath rhythm. If the breath has become shallow or is racing from anxiety or overexertion, this can bring it back into balance, restoring and recovering the breath. Three-part breathing can also be done in an exaggerated way to point out the areas involved as well as any issues in those areas. When lying down, it looks like a wave washing over the body, with one part at a time rising and lowering.

The Practice of Three-Part Breathing
When first learning this, it is helpful to lie down.

- Rest comfortably on your back, either on the floor or in your bed.

- Use a pillow under your head and another under the back of your knees for comfort.

- Place one hand on your lower abdomen below your navel and one hand above your navel on your low ribs.

- As you begin to inhale, expand the abdomen and then the ribs. And as you exhale let the ribs contract and then the abdomen. In other words, let the lower hand rise and then the upper hand as you inhale. As you exhale, let the upper hand lower and then the bottom hand.

- Practice this for several breaths. This is two-part breathing.

- When you have the rhythm, you can add the upper chest. It might be helpful to move the bottom hand to the upper chest below the neck.

- Now as you inhale, expand the abdomen, ribs, and upper chest. As you exhale, contract the upper chest, ribs, and abdomen.

- It will look and feel like a wave as you expand and contract.

- Practice 3–5 times and then let your breath reset and return to a new normal.

- You can return to this practice throughout the day while sitting in a chair as well.

Note: *When three-part breathing becomes easier, you can also experiment with reversing the direction of breath, inhaling as you expand the chest, ribs, and abdomen and exhaling as you contract the abdomen, ribs, and chest. While this is not a natural way to breathe, it provides some flexibility and training for the breath.*

Alternate Nostril Breathing

We have a right nostril breath and a left nostril breath, and our nostril dominance switches from one side to the other throughout the day. We breathe predominantly through one side for somewhere between 60 to 90 minutes and then it switches. The time can vary for each individual, but this switching is always happening.

Bring your attention to your own breathing right now, and you will likely notice that one side is a little more open than the other. It may be very subtle or very obvious. When we have a cold, it is much more apparent. You may have noticed that when you are sick, it seems like the nose is completely blocked on one side and you are just breathing out of one nostril. At some point, you may notice that both nostrils open for a moment and then the dominance switches. The side that was blocked is now open, and the side that was open is now blocked. We just accept it, but have you ever wondered why? The sensitive tissue that lines the nostrils is much like erectile tissue, and it responds by subtly swelling on one side, which blocks the airflow, and then it switches and swells on the other side.

This nasal rhythm is actually connected to the nervous system.[10] The yogis understood this connection and the part it plays in regulating the nervous system. The right nostril has a connection to the sympathetic nervous system, the part of the nervous system responsible for the fight or flight response. It is also responsible for the active functions of the body. It governs heating functions such as digestion, the rise of blood pressure and the pumping action of the heart, and when we are just moving about. The left nostril has a connection to the parasympathetic nervous system, the part of the nervous system responsible for resting and relaxing. It governs cooling functions like the resting phase of the heart and the lowering of blood pressure. The left nostril will naturally open when we are sitting quietly, reading, and listening to music. Both actions of the nervous system are important, as are both phases of the nostril dominance. When we are under stress, that rhythm can get interfered with and confused. For that reason, the practice of alternate nostril breathing helps ensure and protect the natural nasal rhythm.

Additionally, there are times when both nostrils open evenly. One of those times is right before the dominance changes. There is a moment during that change when you can experience this openness. Another time is at sunrise and sunset. This may be surprising, but we are intimately connected to nature and the sun. Without its heat and light we wouldn't be alive. Just like the moon affects a woman's menstrual cycle, the sun affects the breath cycle.

Have you ever been captivated by a sunrise or sunset? When I was vacationing in Door County, Wisconsin, one summer, I noticed how every night at sunset hundreds of people would walk out to the beach and stand looking at the sun, mesmerized by the colors and beauty. As soon as it would set, the crowd would pause and there would be complete silence, and then in the next moment the whole crowd would cheer. I felt like I was part of something special and auspicious. There was a moment of peace that was undeniable. Our nervous system craves this. That is why people take pictures and travel to see the best sunrises and sunsets, to capture the feeling we have when we experience it. That feeling is prompted by a physiological response, one where the nervous system is in a state of balance. It may also be why meditators choose to practice at sunrise and sunset. Not only is there a balance between the light and darkness, but the balance of the nervous system makes the experience of peace palpable. Interestingly enough, another time when the nostrils open evenly is during meditation. So it stands to reason that meditation practitioners would also try to open both nostrils evenly in preparation for meditation to help support the experience.

The practice of alternate nostril breathing helps maintain the fluidity of this process and keeps the shifting rhythm healthy. In addition, it balances the two hemispheres of the brain and the nervous system.

The Practice of Alternate Nostril Breathing—Version I

- Sit comfortably and take a few slow breaths as you relax. Soften your gaze or gently close your eyes.

- Make a loose fist with your right hand. Release the thumb, ring finger, and little finger from the fist. You will use the thumb to close the right nostril at the crease and the little finger and ring finger to close the left nostril at the crease.*

- Inhale slowly and smoothly through both nostrils.

- Use the thumb to close the right nostril at the crease (you don't need much pressure at all, just a light touch will do), and exhale and inhale slowly through the left nostril.

- At the top of that inhale, switch, and use the little finger and ring finger to close the left nostril at the crease. Now exhale and inhale through the right nostril.

- The pattern is exhale, inhale, switch. Exhale, inhale, switch.

- Continue to practice 3 times on each side as you alternate.

- When you finish, release the hand and breathe evenly through both nostrils 3 times. This is 1 round.

- Practice for 1–3 rounds and rest.

* The purpose of this hand position is that the thumb weighs about the same as the little and ring finger combined. This gives equal pressure to each nostril when closing them. Since breathing is such a subtle practice, it is important to approach it with that same subtlety. You may also choose to rest the index and middle finger at the eyebrow center for comfort instead of keeping them in a fist.

The Practice of Alternate Nostril Breathing—Version II

- This version invites you to inhale through both nostrils slowly, then close the right nostril with the right thumb and take three breaths on the left side before switching.

- Close the left nostril with the little finger and ring finger and take three breaths on the right side.

- Allow the breath to be slow, smooth, and quiet.

- When you finish, relax and breathe 3 times through both nostrils evenly.

Note: *Because the tissue in the nose is much like erectile tissue, it can be affected by our thoughts. Try changing your nostril dominance just by thinking about it. If you put your attention to your right nostril with the intention for it to open as the dominant nostril, it will do exactly that. It may take a few minutes, but you have the power to affect this rhythm with just your thoughts. Many meditators will bring their attention to the point between the two nostrils where the upper lip meets the nose bridge. As they do this, they imagine both nostrils opening evenly. This in turn brings the nervous system into balance and prepares the mind for meditation.*

Additionally: *If you struggle with a plugged nose, this exercise can be frustrating and not helpful. In that case, you can work with using your four fingers on your cheek next to your nostril to pull the skin and open the nostril (much like a breathing strip would do). Try it by pulling the skin on one side and taking three slow breaths, then try the other side. Release your hands and imagine breathing evenly through both sides for three more breaths.*

Humming Breath—Bhramari

This is also called the buzzing bee breath. It's done by gently humming or buzzing on the exhalation breath. The buzzing can be done at a pitch that feels calming for you. When I first realized how powerful this practice was, I was walking my fitful three-month-old daughter who was clearly fighting sleep. I noticed that she started making a buzzing sound, and after a few minutes she was sound asleep. It was her way to self-soothe. This sounding is how many babies lull themselves to sleep. Since then I have realized how powerful this practice can be for adults as well. Humming breath helps soothe the nerves, calms and quiets the mind, lowers blood pressure, dissipates anger, and improves restful sleep.

The Practice of Humming Breath

- This practice can be done sitting or lying down.
- Get comfortable, and gently soften your gaze or close your eyes.
- Relax your body.
- Inhale slowly, and as you exhale begin to make a buzzing sound.
- See if you can extend the sound over time. This will help lengthen the exhalation breath.
- Practice anywhere from 3–7 breaths and then be still and quiet. Allow the breath to return to a rhythm that feels easy.

Note: *This practice can also be done by placing the four fingers of each hand over the eyes, while using the thumbs to gently close the ears as you buzz. This can be quite loud internally, so you may need to adjust your sound. It is much more attention grabbing when done this way, and if you are someone who has a busy mind and a frazzled nervous system, this version can be very helpful.*

Breath is one of the quickest and easiest ways to affect stress. Each of these practices can stand alone and be helpful. They can be used in a pinch, or they can be incorporated with your other daily stress management practices. I recommend introducing one or two at a time to use for several weeks and then trying the others in the same way. Once you have worked with them, you may want to choose the ones that are the most supportive for you.

Be open, easy, and curious when you practice. Turning to breath to help you manage stress can be like magic. You can send the breath anywhere that needs energy or healing, and you will notice some release or support in that area. Every inhale breath is life-giving and life-sustaining, while every exhale breath is a moment of peace and surrender.

When we come into this world, the first breath we take is an inspiration. When we leave this world, the last breath we take is an expiration. All the breaths in between are an affirmation that life is precious.

Meditation

Simply Being

"How we regard what arises in meditation is training for how we regard whatever arises in the rest of our lives."
—PEMA CHÖDRÖN[1]

A CENTERING MOMENT
Meditation on Breath

- Sit comfortably in a chair or on the floor.
- Take several long, slow, deep breaths.
- Soften your gaze or close your eyes.
- As you exhale, send a gentle wave of relaxation from top to toe. Take a few of these slow, long breaths as you smooth out any tension within your reach.
- Relax and settle as you begin to seamlessly weave the breaths together.

- Now begin to count your breaths as you exhale. For example, inhale and as you exhale count to yourself "one."

- Continue the count in this way, until you reach the count of 12. When you reach 12, or if you happen to lose track of your count, start over at 1.

- Practice 1–3 rounds of 12 breaths.

- If the mind wanders, notice and simply come back to counting your breaths. When you finish, sit quietly for a few more minutes; when you feel ready, slowly transition back to your day, taking this sense of calm with you.

OFTEN A STUDENT WILL COME UP TO ME AND ANNOUNCE THAT they won't be able to practice meditation because they can't make their mind "blank." My response is always the same: "Thank goodness for that, because if your mind was blank, you wouldn't be alive." Often a look of confusion follows. Somehow the notion that meditation is the practice of making the mind blank, or even stopping the mind, has become a common assumption, but the mind is always moving. We can't stop it, but we *can* hope for the ability to rise above or settle beneath the constant rumbling of thoughts in the mind.

Seldom do we realize how busy the mind is until we try to sit still. When we are moving, we're less likely to notice the way our minds jump from thought to thought. As we sit still with our thoughts, it can feel like the mind is getting busier, but the truth is that it's always busy; we just don't notice it as much when we are moving with it. We run all day from one thing to the next, and the minute we sit still, the mind starts to unwind or in some cases ruminate. This often contributes to those sleepless nights, when we just can't seem to turn our minds off. If we don't have a process for letting go of some of these thoughts and feelings, they can build up and the mind becomes impossible to settle.

The practice of meditation helps us calm and process this never-ending stream of thoughts. It involves both concentration and what is called "passive attentiveness." In passive attentiveness, we start to pay attention to whatever is arising in the mind, while letting go of any attachment to those thoughts. Simply put, we let the thoughts arise and dissipate without labeling them or judging them, without getting lost in the story or the drama. We step back and gently observe, and then let them go. In time and with practice, the mind begins to settle. If we stop feeding thoughts, they eventually stop coming up with the same velocity. What seemed like a tsunami is now slow, gentle waves. In deeper states of meditation, the mind may become like a clear pond with just an occasional ripple.

In order to observe thought without getting pulled in, the mind needs some sort of anchor, a point of focus. Practicing focused attention or concentration is what leads to the experience of meditation. By gathering the attention and allowing it to rest on your chosen point of focus or an object, we are giving the mind somewhere to rest.

In the meditative traditions of Yoga and Buddhism, they talk about the mind being busy like a monkey, and they refer to the mind in meditation as a "monkey mind." I never understood this analogy until I went to India. It was so interesting to see the monkeys wandering freely everywhere. The street vendors would put ropes in the trees next to their goods because when the monkeys are left with nothing to do, they wreak havoc on the vendors' goods. One way to calm a monkey is to give it a rope. If a monkey sees a rope, it will go up and down the rope all day rather than rushing from thing to thing in a frenetic way. At one point while I was shopping, I looked up and there was a monkey hanging from a rope over my head. It was happily swinging while the street was bustling with shoppers. In the same way, if you give the mind an object to rest on, it will become deliberate, quiet, and calm. The breath, a mantra, a prayer, and a candle flame are just a few ways to give the monkey mind a rope.

When we meditate, we train ourselves to step back and witness without adding to the drama and chaos of our own thought process. By stepping back, thoughts and feelings begin to lose their power over us, and we begin to see things differently. We have the space to observe the nature of what is arising in us and then choose how we want to react or respond. We aren't caught in the loop of our reactions. This begins to translate into our lives when we experience an uncomfortable emotion or an upsetting thought, and we are able to look at it from a more rational and spacious perspective rather than automatically assuming and reacting. Then we are empowered to choose our own way of responding, and we stop feeling like a victim of our circumstances, thoughts, and feelings. This practice builds tolerance and patience.

When you practice meditation, you will begin to notice that things that used to bother you just don't seem to bother you in the same way. This is one of the greatest gifts of meditation. When working with cardiac patients, we often refer to this by saying that "your fuse gets longer." Everyone can relate to that. How many times have you snapped at someone or lost your cool about something that you later regret?

The greatest joy for me as a teacher of meditation is to see the changes in students from week to week. Their faces look more relaxed, they smile more, and move with less urgency. They carry themselves with a sense of ease that is evident and irrefutable. While your own personal experience of meditation is the most reliable evidence for its importance, the research on meditation alone is mounting, and practicing some form of meditation daily can be key to managing stress and improving overall health and well-being.

Several studies have pointed to the fact that meditation plays a key role in reducing stress that can cause inflammation, oxidative stress, plaque formation, and heart disease.[2] Even the American Heart Association suggests that meditation can be considered an adjunct to cardiovascular risk reduction interventions.[3] This is not surprising, but rather a clear indication that the power of meditation should not be overlooked in the prevention and treatment of cardiovascular disease. Since the practice of meditation is safe and the impact substantial, it naturally leads to more interest on the part of those suffering from the effects of stress on heart health to take more responsibility for their own healing.

While there are many ways to practice meditation, and some of the studies cite different types and techniques of meditation practice, research shows that "all types of meditation are associated with blood pressure control, enhancement in insulin resistance, reduction of lipid peroxidation and cellular senescence, independent of the type of meditation."[4] Since there are several meditation techniques to choose from, this is great news, allowing individuals to pick the technique that best fits their particular temperament and nature.

At the core, most meditation techniques share the common practice of bringing the mind to rest on a point of focus, or what is called an "object for meditation." Asking the mind to rest on anything can be challenging, since the mind has an infinite number of directions it can travel through free association.

There are two choices when looking for a place to let the mind rest in meditation. One is something outside of you, or an external object, and another is something within, or an internal object. What works for one person may not work for another. We all have our unique differences, and it's important to recognize those differences even when choosing a meditation technique. We each have predispositions and lifestyle habits that make choosing a meditation technique an important process. No matter what you choose, it's helpful if that object feels uplifting and you feel a connection to it.

MEDITATION TECHNIQUES UTILIZING EXTERNAL OBJECTS
Meditation on a Candle Flame or Image

An example of an external object might be a candle flame, a flower, or a beautiful image like a landscape. If you don't have a beautiful view out your window for meditation, you could use a picture of a beautiful view. Sometimes, I go through old travel magazines and look for amazing images to use. Even an image on your computer screen works well. Special stones or shells that inspire a sense of peace or joy can also be used as an object to facilitate the experience of meditation.

This practice involves gazing at an external object and focusing attention on it until you feel the urge to close your eyes and draw that image into your mind or your heart. Once the image fades, gently open your eyes and rest them again on the external object. Here you are straddling both the external world and internal world as you practice. This practice can be very calming and soothing.

This practice may best fit those who:

- Prefer keeping the eyes open or who feel fear when closing the eyes.
- Tend to fall asleep in meditation with their eyes closed.
- Require a tangible transition from the activities of the day.
- Feel uplifted and inspired by the beauty around them.

Candle-Gazing Meditation

- Sit quietly in front of a candle flame (it's helpful to trim the wick first).
- Begin to relax the body by sending a wave of relaxation from top to toe.
- Now open your eyes, and with a soft gaze, let your attention rest on the candle flame.

- Hold your awareness to the flame; you may notice the size, color, and movement.

- When you grow tired of holding your gaze, close your eyes and imagine drawing the flame inward, to the center of your eyebrows or into the center of your heart. Choose whatever location feels right to you.

- Hold the flame there until it disappears, or you can't hold it any longer.

- Gently open your eyes again and gaze at the candle flame.

- Repeat this several times, allowing the duration of your attention outward and inward to lengthen if possible. It may even feel good to keep the eyes closed a little longer. Listen to your own body and follow its lead.

- When you feel ready, gently complete the practice and relax the eyes.

- Cup your hands and bring them over your eyes. Notice how you feel.

- Release your hands and transition back to activity slowly.

Walking Meditation

In walking meditation the focus is on the slow movement of your footsteps connecting to the earth each time you take a step. It is done with your eyes open and your attention resting with each step you take. The breath and mind begin to slow down and come into a rhythm.

This practice may best fit those who:

- Have a hard time sitting still.
- Don't want to close their eyes to meditate.
- Need a physical practice to help them settle down.

- Are inspired by taking in their surroundings in a contemplative way.

Walking meditation can be done barefoot or with shoes. When done barefoot, it helps bring synovial fluid into the joints of the feet. The feet have many bones and joints, and walking barefoot helps keep the joints juicy, which in turn supports better balance.

Find an open, quiet area either inside or outside (if practicing outside, be aware of the elements; if it is too sunny or hot, it may be best to choose a shaded area).

- Grab a wrist behind your back or let the arms hang gently down alongside your body.
- Unlock your knees and feel the feet contacting the earth.
- Now notice a gentle and effortless lift to the spine.
- The gaze of the eyes is downward, but the chin and spine stay lifted throughout the practice.
- Pick up one foot and place it gently in front of you. Slowly commit the weight to that foot.
- Now pick up the other foot and slowly step forward and then shift the weight.
- As you walk, become aware of the connection of the feet to the earth and the shifting weight.
- Try to keep a pace that allows you to move without wavering. This pace is different for everyone.
- At first you may walk with a little more speed, until you get the hang of it.
- Once you feel more balanced, you can try to slow your pace and let the breath find a natural rhythm.
- Little by little, slow your pace.

- Practice anywhere from 5–15 minutes.
- When finished, be still for a moment and take in the stillness. You can sit or stand for this.
- Transition back to activity slowly.

Mindfulness

Bringing your full attention to what you are doing while you are doing it is called mindfulness.[5] When eating food or doing daily tasks, bringing a one-pointed awareness to your every action is a way to not only improve awareness but also bridge the gap between the world outside you and the world within.

Another way mindfulness is used is during meditation. In meditation we bring full attention to an object (breath, candle, mantra, etc.), and when the mind wanders or drifts, we pause and mindfully notice where the attention has gone. Without labeling or judging, without ruminating or getting lost in the drama, we simply come back, returning the attention to the point of focus. This act of observing where the attention goes is also called mindfulness.

This practice may best fit those who:

- Find multitasking overwhelming to the mind.
- Need a transition from work or activities.
- Want to bridge the tasks of everyday life with the internal practice of meditation.

Mindful Eating Practice

Mindfulness practice can be done with just about any daily task, such as taking a shower, sweeping the floor, doing the dishes, and so on. Here I have chosen to discuss eating since there are some positive effects of mindful eating that help improve digestion and nutrition. We all eat every day, and using a mindfulness exercise, even with just the first few bites of food, can have a profound impact on digestive health and overall well-being.

- Sit with your food in front of you and gently close your eyes.
- Take a few deep breaths and begin to take in the aromas of the food.
- As you open your eyes, gaze gently upon the food, and notice the textures and colors.
- Begin to imagine all the people involved in growing the food. Imagine the people who picked it, those who brought it to you, and those who prepared it for you.
- Then imagine the elements involved in supporting that growth—the earth and soil, the rain and water, the sun, and the air.
- Now as you take your first bite, just hold it on your tongue for a moment and notice the aromas and flavors. As salivation begins, chew the food slowly and let it dissolve almost to liquid before swallowing. Pause a moment to take in all the sensations and flavors.
- Let the foods you are eating nourish your body and mind.
- Take the next several bites with this kind of awareness and attention to the act of chewing and swallowing.
- Linger in this presence and unity with your food.
- You can practice with the first few bites or try it with your entire meal.

MEDITATION TECHNIQUES UTILIZING AN INTERNAL OBJECT
Breath-Centered Meditation
When we breathe, the breath flows in two directions. By letting our attention rest on this rhythmic flow of breath as it comes and goes, we can gather and focus our attention. As we begin to

breathe, it soothes and calms the nervous system. We always have our breath with us, and for this reason it makes it an easy choice for a meditation technique.

This practice may best fit those who:

- Find the rhythm of breath soothing and grounding.
- Are overworked or under a lot of stress.
- Experience too much stimulation.
- Are prone to anxiety.

Note: In some cases of anxiety or for those who have asthma or other breathing issues, it may be too unsettling to let the attention rest on an irregular breath rhythm. In this case choosing one of the other meditation techniques may be a better place to start.

- Sit comfortably in a chair or on the floor.
- Begin to settle into the space your body occupies.
- Notice the connection of your sitting bones to the chair or floor beneath you.
- Now find an easy, effortless lift of your spine.
- Send a gentle wave of relaxation throughout your body.
- As the body settles and relaxes, become aware of your breathing.
- Let the breath find its own natural rhythm.
- Begin to notice the breath in the nostrils.
- Plant your attention on the breath entering and leaving the body through the nostrils.
- Ride the breath like a wave. Stay with it as it comes in and as it goes out.

- Let your breath stay in the foreground of your awareness while all thoughts and sensations, emotions and impressions settle to the background.

- As thoughts and feelings come to the foreground, notice, and without labeling or judging, without analyzing or ruminating, gently return your attention to the breath.

- Continue returning to the breath when the mind drifts or wanders, toggling between mindfully observing whatever is arising and your attention to the breath.

- Practice for a few minutes on your own.

- When finished, make a smooth transition back to your activities.

Meditation on a Word, Prayer, or Mantra

This type of meditation involves letting the mind rest on a word, short prayer, or mantra that is repeated in the mind or heart. This technique is interwoven with mindfulness so that when thoughts and feelings arise, they are held and observed without judgment. As we observe thoughts without judging, we can begin to let go of them. It is then that the mind can gently return to its focus and rest.

Not everyone has a connection to a religious tradition, but if you do and you want to bridge that with your meditation practice, you can use a prayer from that tradition as your meditation object.

This practice may best fit those who:

- Feel connected to their religious/spiritual tradition and want to bridge meditation with their spiritual life.

- Need the support of a sound to hold the attention inward.

Note: *Before you begin, reflect on a word, prayer, sound, or mantra that you feel connected to, something that brings you a sense of peace or calm.*

If using a prayer, it's best if it is a short prayer that invokes a connection to the source. If using a word, let it be uplifting.

- Sit either on the floor or in a chair. If on the floor, use a cushion under the sitting bones to lift the spine and take some pressure off the low back and hips.
- Begin to settle as you find the connection of the sitting bones to the floor or chair.
- Find an effortless inner lift to your spine.
- Now take several slow, deep breaths as you begin to soften and relax.
- Allow the gaze of your eyes to soften downward, or gently close your eyes.
- Bring your attention to the center of your chest (the heart center) or the point between your eyebrows (the eyebrow center). Choose what feels natural to you.
- Start to notice your breathing, without changing it.
- Begin to internally repeat the mantra, prayer, or word without uttering a sound and without moving the lips. Let the sound draw you inward.
- The sound doesn't need to be in sync with the breath. If it flows with the breath, allow it, and if it doesn't flow, let it be.
- Try to accept whatever arises in the body or mind with equanimity.
- Recognize if you are judging, analyzing, or ruminating and try to let go.
- When the mind drifts off—and it will—gently come back to your chosen mantra or prayer and rest your attention on that.

- Continue to toggle between one pointed attention to your chosen object and mindful awareness of whatever is arising in the mind and body.

- At some point in the practice, you may find yourself losing interest in thoughts. Simply allow yourself to settle deeper into stillness and presence.

- When you are ready to come out (5–20 minutes), begin to deepen the in breath and lengthen the out breath. Gently open your eyes or raise your gaze. Transition slowly.

Note: *With time and practice, you may notice that if you pause while repeating the sound, you can still hear it like an echo. You may want to pause and listen from time to time. When your attention drifts, continue repeating it.*

Meditation on a Feeling

This is a practice that calls us inward, using a feeling to anchor the attention. We recall a feeling that is uplifting and creates a sense of deep joy or peace. We hold that feeling in the heart and rest in it. When it fades, we return to that feeling and let it fill the heart again.

This practice may best fit those who:

- Want to access emotions.

- Easily access feelings and want to transcend them.

- Spend a lot of time in the mind and would like to balance thinking with feeling.

Before you begin, remember a time when you felt a sense of deep joy. It may have been when you were with someone you love, like a grandparent, child, or grandchild, or even a pet. It may have been a time when you were in nature or traveling. It could be a time you were actively having fun at an amusement park or enjoying a concert. Take a moment and trust whatever comes to you.

- Sit comfortably in a chair or on the floor.
- Take a few slow, deep breaths.
- Begin to recall a time when you felt deep joy.
- Let your mind connect to the memory and the feelings that are associated with that memory.
- Notice the changes in your body and in your mind. The memory may even bring a smile to your face.
- Stay with that feeling of joy. Let it fill your heart and mind.
- Let go of the memory and stay with the feeling.
- When the feeling fades, return to it. If you need to, you can return to the memory again to remember the feeling. Continue in this way, using the feeling of joy as your anchor in meditation.
- One part of your awareness is resting in the feeling of joy, and another part is bearing witness to whatever is arising in the mind.
- When you are ready (5–20 minutes), begin to deepen your breathing. Open your eyes or raise your gaze. Take your time to transition.

SETTING UP A DAILY MEDITATION PRACTICE
Finding Time
When setting up a meditation practice, there is always the issue of time. One of the first things people say when confronted with the question of time is "I don't have the time for meditation."

I used to respond by saying, "You don't have the time *not* to practice meditation," but that felt too esoteric and not helpful. The truth is that we create time for what we feel is important. We create time to brush our teeth, eat, sleep, watch the news, scroll through social media, read, and talk to friends.

We build time into our lives for what seems essential. So the real issue is seeing meditation and a daily stress management practice as essential and important. I can tell you how important these practices are to your health and that might inspire you for a short time, but if you don't experience it as beneficial, you won't make time for it.

So the first thing to consider is a commitment to a trial period. Do it regularly for one month. No excuses. It's helpful to keep a journal to notice how you feel each day you practice. It's also helpful to find external support when your internal stamina waivers. We can't always remember what is good for us in times of stress and chaos. That's when we might turn to the support of others to help inspire us when we need reinforcement. Inviting friends or family members to join you in a meditation practice can be one way to create a support system. Joining an online meditation group or a local meditation group in your area is yet another way to maintain a daily habit.

The practices of relaxation and meditation may require an investment of your time each day, but what they give you in return is deep and profound. In addition, you may notice feeling calmer as you flow through your days with greater ease.

Meditation puts us "in the zone." We don't seem to spin our wheels and we get a lot done in a little bit of time because we are focused and relaxed. It helps us work smarter and manage our time without all the frenetic energy.

When I worked with heart patients as part of an integrative team, our whole team knew that doing these daily practices was essential for patient outcomes and heart health. We all saw the results over and over again even when patients didn't have faith in the practice. When patients would say, "I can't fit this into my busy life," our response was always the same: "Don't try to fit meditation into your life, allow your life to take shape around your meditation practices." If you put these stress management practices first, your life and health will take shape around them. In other words, make them essential and you won't have to think about constantly fitting them in. You probably don't think about fitting your shower or toothbrushing into your day. You just do it because it's essential.

How Much Time Do I Need?

I often hear meditation teachers say things like, "Even just a couple minutes a day is helpful." And while in theory that sounds good, the reality is that in those first several minutes of meditation the mind is just unwinding the thoughts and concerns of the day. You may hear the latest jingle still making its way through the mind, or you may still be working out all the interactions of the day. If we don't give ourselves a little time for these to unwind and dissipate, we won't move beyond them, into a deeper state of being.

That said, if you can dedicate 15 to 30 minutes once or twice a day, you will allow some time for the thoughts to unwind and the natural rhythm of meditation to emerge. If you have a regular daily practice, taking a few minutes to return to meditation throughout the day can link you to your deeper practice fairly quickly, and then there is some benefit from those short sessions throughout the day.

Some people like to set a timer or chime to remind them when the time is up. You could even place a small clock or watch next to you to help you keep track of time, rather than spending your meditation practice wondering how long it has been or how much time you have left to go.

What Time of Day Is Best

The best time of day to practice is always when you have the time and space. Early in the morning, before dinner, or before bed can be natural times in the day when a space opens up. Early in the morning, the mind is fresh and rested, so it may be easier to concentrate. The practice can help you get centered and balanced before your day starts. Later in the day, after work and before dinner, it can help you transition from your day and free the mind of excess clutter so you can enter your evening unburdened and clear. Meditation before bed can help release any held tension from the day and allow you to make a graceful transition into a deep and restful sleep. Ultimately a practice should align with your own rhythm and schedule, so it serves you and your patterns. Once you find a time, do your best to honor it each day so it can become a habit.

Creating Space

Each room in your house has an energy pattern. What happens in a room creates an energy pattern that subtly affects our own energy field. When I am in my office, my mind is especially busy and task-focused, but when I leave, my mind gets quieter. It's true of meditation as well. If we practice in the same place, we create energy that lingers in that place. If you can carve out a place for meditation in your own home, it will call you back to the practice each time you walk by. It's like a faint whisper that in time gets louder. Some people like to place meaningful or sacred objects in their meditation space to infuse it with a quality that calls them inward. Using pictures of loved ones, a candle, a journal, pictures of inspiring teachers, or poetry can make it feel more inviting. Others prefer a clean and simple open space that calls them into that feeling of openness. Whatever calls you to practice is best.

Picking a Seated Posture

So many images of meditation involve someone sitting on the floor with the legs crossed and spine straight. It's not that this isn't a good position for some; it's just that it can be very off-putting for those who can't sit that way comfortably.

For many of us, it may be more helpful to sit in a chair or find a position on the floor with support under the sitting bones and perhaps under the knees. Even sitting against a wall can help support the back. If you want to try sitting on the floor, start by playing with a stack of pillows and finding a position that not only feels easy on your joints, but is also steady and stable. I like to sit on a small ottoman since it is a little lower to the ground and I feel comfortable. It's a position where I can easily sit upright.

Since meditation involves passive attention, sitting upright keeps the mind alert and less likely to drift into sleep. It's helpful to settle into the sitting bones and let gravity ground the body. This sets a nice foundation for passive attention and stillness. In this position, the spine is free to gently lift up out of the pelvis. Once you have found a steady and comfortable pose, there are a few other things to consider as well to set yourself up for success.

The mind tends to take the path of the extremities. The hands want to grasp, and the feet want to move. And this restlessness affects the mind in meditation. One way to quiet the mind is to use a mudra, or a hand position that seals and directs energy. One that is very effective is done by gently joining the thumb and index finger on each hand, pressing them lightly together like you are holding a piece of hair or silk thread between them. Not only does this redirect the energy that is traveling out through the fingers back inward, but it also lets you know that the mind has wandered off when the seal is broken.

Another practice that can be helpful is to sit cross-legged. This is a way to seal the energy that wants to move out with the feet and redirect that energy back inward. Not everyone can sit with the legs crossed, however, so another way to create this is to cover the feet or, if sitting on a chair, cross the ankles.

Additionally, it helps to cover the body with a shawl or blanket. This creates a bit of barrier from the external world, and it redirects the attention inward. It can also keep you warm, since meditation lowers blood pressure and the body may feel cold as a result.

Finding Your Own Meditation Practice

All these suggestions can help make the transition to meditation smoother and easier. Another way to transition into meditation is by practicing gentle movements, relaxation, and breathing as taught in the previous chapters. These practices can serve to romance the mind into meditation. They are designed to deliver you to the doorstep of meditation so that the transition is seamless. When you weave the practices together in this way, it feels as if you have arrived in the experience of meditation with little or no effort.

When meditation is practiced without the preparation of postures, relaxation, and breathing, it may require a little more effort to prepare yourself. In that case, I will often spend a few minutes relaxing and breathing before I begin the practice. Using a short practice of centering from chapter 3 and a brief practice of alternate nostril breathing from chapter 4 can be a helpful way to step into meditation.

Every meditation technique has value, and the one that works best for you may not be the best for someone else. Some people find that blending the techniques works best. They might use a candle-gazing meditation and, as the mind calms down, transition to a breath-centered meditation. Others start with following the breath and use a prayer or mantra once the breath has come into a quiet rhythm. There are no rules, yet once you find a technique that works, it's helpful to stay with it so it can take you deeper. There is an ancient proverb that says, "You can't reach water if you dig a bunch of shallow wells." In the same way, you can't know the depths of meditation if you don't dig deep. Staying with one technique for a period of time will lead you to the depths of your own being in profound and powerful ways.

We spend much of the day cluttering our minds with unnecessary thoughts and impressions. We scroll social media, look at screens, and take in all kinds of sensory input. We are constantly processing the world around us. Taking a few minutes to unplug and let it all settle is vital. Our minds and nervous system require downtime now more than ever before. We need to be still. We need a daily digital detox program, and meditation is the answer.

Not only does meditation help us unplug, but it strengthens our ability to hold our own stories. We start by sitting with a willingness to be with whatever we have been pushing away, whatever scares us. What we suppress and push down has a way of coming back up to the surface to be healed. If we ignore it or push it back down, it can make us sick or keep us stuck. If we allow it to surface and let it be expressed without our usual reactions, it starts to unwind. We allow our inner stories to be exposed without pushing them away or pulling them in. We develop the courage to be present with ourselves just as we are. We find an unwavering strength in the face of adversity.

When we are determined to sit with our own stories with openness, courage, and equanimity, our patience and tolerance begin to expand. We develop compassion and understanding for ourselves and others. Our minds and our lives become more spacious, and we can see ourselves with more clarity. A feeling of unity and belonging replaces our sense of separateness and isolation. Meditation connects us to our inner world and brings a sense of meaning and clarity to our lives. It creates the balance that lets us live in harmony with ourselves and others.

Imagery

A Healing Shift

"We are what we pretend to be, so we must be careful about what we pretend to be."

—Kurt Vonnegut Jr.[1]

A Centering Moment

Imagine Healing Your Heart

- Begin by sitting in a chair or lying on the floor.
- Gently close your eyes.
- Take several slow, deep breaths and begin to relax.
- Begin resting your awareness in the spaces of your own heart.
- Imagine how your heart looks, how it feels, how it sounds.
- Now breathe as if your own heart could breathe.

- Imagine the breath creating a spaciousness and sense of freedom in and around your heart.

- Knowing that the mind controls the muscles that surround the artery walls, begin to envision the artery walls relaxing. Observe the blood and energy flowing with graceful ease to and from the heart. See it in the mind's eye and feel the flow in and around the heart.

- Imagine all areas of the heart free from blockages both physical and emotional. Even if you can't see it or feel it clearly, imagine that you do.

- Gently hold onto that feeling. Rest in that for several breaths.

- Connect to the powerful healing shift that is happening right now.

- Place that feeling in your cellular memory and return to it anytime.

- When you feel ready, make a gentle transition. Raise your gaze and open your eyes.

WE OFTEN UNDERESTIMATE THE CAPACITY OF OUR OWN IMAGI-nation, but how we imagine ourselves plays a major role in who we are and what we become. Our thoughts have a powerful role in shaping our lives. The held beliefs we have about ourselves can either lift us up or keep us in patterns that don't allow us to realize our fullest potential.

Imagery can be used to invoke a healing response within the body and mind, and this practice is being used widely as an intervention to empower patients in their own self-care, giving them a feeling of control and autonomy around their own healing process.[2] A 2020 study states: "Guided imagery is a therapeutic approach that has been used for centuries. Through the use of mental imagery, the mind-body connection is activated to enhance an individual's sense of well-being and reduce stress and anxiety. It has the ability to enhance the individual's immune system. There is research and data to support the use of guided imagery for patient outcomes."[3] Because of this scientific support, this ancient technique is now becoming a part of many integrative care practices and continues to be used in many aspects of health and healing.

If you are wondering how your thoughts can affect your physiology, try this exercise. Begin to imagine a big, juicy lemon. Now, envision cutting it open and seeing the juice dripping as you take the knife and cut a small sliver. See yourself placing the lemon wedge against your tongue. Taste the juice of the lemon in your mouth as you bite into it. At this point you can probably feel yourself salivating and maybe even puckering at the simple thought of eating a lemon. Your imagination just caused a physiological response. What we imagine can and does have a powerful effect on our body and mind.

We are always using imagery. If imagery seems illusive, ask yourself, "Have you ever worried about anything?" The usual response starts with a tentative laugh, "Of course, and I'm pretty good at that." Just the simple practice of worry is a form of imagery. It's a negative form that can have consequences for our health and well-being, but if we turn it around it can also help us achieve good health as well as realize our goals. How we talk to ourselves and how we think about ourselves is key to our own healing.

Worry itself can set off a cascade of physical symptoms that can chip away at our health and well-being. I know it wouldn't take much for you to remember a time when worry raised your blood pressure or upset your stomach or even ruined your day. When one of my daughters was learning to drive, I can easily recall a detailed "awfulization" experience that made me feel sick.

I gave my sixteen-year-old daughter Gracie the keys to the car and asked her to be home by 11:00 p.m. At 11:10 p.m. I tried to call, but no answer. I sent a frantic text. Nothing. From there the awfulizing began. I had heard stories of teens who had been in terrible car accidents shortly after getting a driver's license. The details of these circumstances are enough to make any mother's heart ache with grief. Just recalling any part of that scenario is devastating. In just a short time, my heart was racing, my palms were sweating, my mouth was dry, and the room began to spin. At 11:20 p.m. the phone rang, "Hi Mom, I fell asleep watching TV with friends, I'm on my way home now. Sorry." I took a deep sigh of relief, but for the next 30 to 40 minutes, I was still processing the adrenaline circulating in my system (it takes at least that long for those stress hormones to come back into balance). The reaction I had didn't help the current situation, of course, and it certainly wouldn't have been helpful if there really was a problem to respond to.

Over time, this kind of response takes a toll on the body. If negative imagery can cause a physiological response, then how does imagining a positive outcome affect us? Even if we can't change an outcome, positive imagery can help us change the way we respond to that outcome.

TURNING AROUND NEGATIVE IMAGERY

If "awfulizing" can affect the body in negative ways, consider that visualizing a positive outcome can truly have a positive impact on your health and well-being. At the very least you can save yourself the wear and tear on your own body that occurs from worry and negative thinking. This doesn't mean that you should avoid difficult situations or try to imagine them away. There is value in being present to situations and letting ourselves be with "what is," without the push or pull of wanting it to be different. Sometimes the right path is to settle into the experience and feel what we need to feel when we need to feel it. Meditation can help us with this process of being present and willing to sit with whatever comes our way. Imagery is not an escape from our feelings or our lives;

it's a way to manage a mind that has the tendency to go off the rails and lead us into unnecessary suffering. It is also a way to use the power of the mind in our own best interests.

When you find your mind going down the path of negative imagery, it's helpful to pause and begin to cultivate the opposite position. The more you are able to polish this skill of shifting from a negative image to a positive one, the more you will be able to shape the outcomes in your own life. In the tradition of yoga this shifting is called Pratipaksha Bhavana. In Sanskrit, *pratipaksha* means "opposite" and *bhavana* means "cultivation," in essence turning a negative into a positive, or the willingness to tell a different story by feeding the story we want to manifest. Much of the stress we suffer from is self-created. It is a consequence of the way we frame what is happening. With this practice, you can begin to retrain the mind to think more positively and reduce the suffering that comes with negative thought patterns and negative imagery.

My partner is a psychotherapist, and much of his work is helping people reframe and re-envision themselves and what they are capable of. It's the job of the therapist to hold a vision of what's possible for each person until they can see it themselves. Sometimes it's hard for us to maintain a vision of what's possible. We can lose sight of ourselves in all the chaos and confusion of everyday life. Imagery can provide clarity and direction. It can lift us up and help us remember who we are and what is possible.

Most of what we accomplish in life starts as a goal or vision that we reach by being able to imagine ourselves manifesting that vision. When working to imagine a positive outcome, we might reimagine a situation we are struggling with and begin to change the narrative by cultivating an opposite perspective. In addition to reframing to imagine a positive outcome, there are other ways to work with imagery, including specific imagery, non-specific imagery, and intention setting.

During specific imagery, we connect directly to the area of the body that needs healing.

Our organs have consciousness, and we can connect to that consciousness through imagery. We can specifically imagine our organs or other parts of the body and mind healing. In the case of non-specific imagery, we can imagine ourselves in a calm place and a serene state so the body and mind can relax and heal. In this way, we use our imagination indirectly to heal the body or mind.

Lastly, with intention setting, there is a goal or intention that is imagined and held in the mind's eye during a calm and centered moment. This intention is returned to over and over to help it take shape in our lives, like planting a seed and watering it so it will grow. With imagery the opportunities are endless. We aren't bound by the physical world, and we can move into a world that allows us to expand into what normally may seem impossible and bring it to a place of possibility.

Imagery and meditation work together. While meditation allows us to focus our attention, imagery then helps us direct it. Meditation is like the magnifying glass we used as kids to harness the light of the sun and burn paper. Imagery is akin to moving that fire around on the paper and burning a design of our choosing. Meditation helps us harness the energy, and imagery sends it wherever we direct it.

As you enter the world of imagery, allow the stories and images offered by your own imagination to begin to illuminate your own excitement and understanding of the importance of using the mind to create positive change in your immediate situation. The suggested images are just a starting point from which to journey into the immense possibilities of using the mind to explore healing and happiness.

SPECIFIC IMAGERY

In the practice of specific imagery, you conjure a healing image that is specific to you and your own health and well-being. You might imagine a clogged artery opening up, or better blood flow to and from the heart. One person I worked with was a programmer, and he used to imagine going into his arteries and seeing the plaque that was there and then hitting the "delete" button on his computer, at which point all the plaque would disappear. He would then imagine the blood flowing freely to and from his heart. I like that image and often use some version of it myself when I want pain or discomfort in an area to disappear.

Another person, a local artist who worked in neon, would imagine brightly colored neon bubbling through his arteries and clearing away any unwanted obstructions. He said he would change the color depending on what healing felt like to him that day. Another man who was living in the United States, away from his family in England, used to imagine his sisters inside his arteries sweeping away the plaque for him. He said he missed the care and love that they showed him for so many years, and he felt closer to them when he did this practice. I used to catch him smiling with delight when he practiced.

One of my favorite imagery examples comes from one of the yoga therapists I know. She had an older man in her program, and he loved spending time with his many grandchildren. During his imagery practice, he would imagine them all at a water park at the top of a series of long and winding waterslides. He would see and feel them screaming with joy as they flew down the slides as if they were in his own heart, clearing a pathway from his arteries to his heart with water splashing everywhere. Not only did this bring him joy, but he felt and truly believed it was cleaning his arteries of unwanted plaque.

For some people, it can be helpful to use an actual scan of the area affected so they can imagine with more precision and clarity. The more personal and relevant you can make the image, the more powerful the effect it can have. It's important to make it fun and personal, and as creative as you are comfortable with. It's with this image that you are telling yourself anything is possible. The limitations in this practice are of your own making. The mind has such an infinite wisdom and range of possibility. You are the only one stopping you. And you are the one who can be involved in your own healing imagery. Of course, if your image feels unattainable it will interfere with your ability to believe and manifest your intent. You can always go bigger once you start to trust the process and your ability to affect your own healing.

Early in my work with heart patients, we would tell them to imagine an artery that was blocked now opening. After some of the initial scans came back, they indicated changes in the areas where the patients were using imagery. The thing we didn't expect was that now other arteries looked more blocked. There was nothing we could really attribute this to, so we started asking patients to use their imagery more broadly, imagining the arteries opening and then all the arteries opening and healing. It was never clear what was happening with those scans, but it didn't matter. We just decided that it's easy to imagine, so go for it. Think big and heal everything, extending the power of imagery to create a healing shift in any and all areas that are in need.

Specific Imagery Practice I

This can be done anywhere you feel safe and comfortable. Closing your eyes can help support an internal image, but if closing your eyes feels uncomfortable you can try this with your eyes softly open and relaxed.

If you have an actual image like an X-ray or scan, you can look at that image for a few moments before you begin to imagine it. Otherwise, imagine it to the best of your ability in your mind's eye. For the sake of this practice I am using the heart as the specific area in need of healing, but you can imagine any other area or organ specific to your own experience.

- Lie on the floor or sit in a chair. Allow yourself to get comfortable.
- Begin to relax the body by sending the breath like a wave from top to toe. Smooth out any tension that is within

your reach. Let go of any tension you are willing and able to let go of.

- Close your eyes and call into your awareness an area in your own body or mind that is in need of healing.

- Imagine it and what it looks like to the best of your ability in your mind's eye.

- Now imagine that there is a small chest of healing tools sitting close to you. Inside this chest are the tools you will need to heal yourself right now. Imagine opening the chest and looking inside. As you dig through the different tools, choose one that calls out to you. It could be something real or imagined—a realistic image or a cartoon image or even something that you have never seen before. Gently pick it up and imagine yourself using it to heal yourself.

- Begin to see and feel this area healing. If it's an artery that is blocked, you might imagine that the blockage is dissolving, and the blood and energy are able to move freely to and from the heart.

- Notice any signs or sensations of healing. This could be a warm or tingling sensation. It's okay if there is no sensation; be assured, it is still working.

- If it's an area that is in pain, you may imagine the pain dissolving. Whatever it is, design the imagery practice for your specific situation. Remember, you can color outside the lines. Make this yours, and bring as much detail to the imagery practice as you can imagine. Let it be specific to you.

- Stay with this practice for as long as you feel connected. Be willing to change and shift if the image transforms in some way. (For example, you may start by imagining sweeping the plaque in your arteries with a broom, and then the broom becomes a vacuum cleaner that sucks up the plaque in the hard-to-reach areas, and finally you may enlist a magic wand to dissolve any remaining plaque and heal any additional areas that need healing. Be creative and remember that in the world of imagination, anything is possible.)

- Be still and sense the healing shift. Rest in that for a few moments.
- Allow your experience of healing to be deep and profound.
- Make a slow and gentle transition when you have finished.

Specific Imagery Practice II (Healing Light)

- Begin by sitting or lying down.
- Soften your gaze and close your eyes.
- Take a few conscious, slow, deep breaths.
- Let your whole body relax.
- Begin to imagine a healing light or healing energy sitting just above the top of your head. It can be light of any color that feels healing, or energy of any vibration that feels healing.
- Hold your attention to the light or energy and let it get brighter and stronger.
- Imagine drawing it into the body through the top of the head and sending it over the mind, healing the mind. Send healing down the spine and through to the vital organs. Down the arms to the fingers, down the legs to the toes.
- Allow it to touch every fiber of your being.
- Now direct that healing to any specific areas that are in need of healing.
- Hold it in those areas, one area at a time, and let the light or energy get brighter and stronger, creating a powerful healing transformation.

- Know that something deep inside has shifted, and let yourself align with this shift.
- When you have finished, slowly open your eyes and transition.

Sharing Images with Others

When you practice imagery, it can be helpful to share your images with others who practice. Talk about them, and ask what others are doing to heal themselves. This helps broaden your own self-imposed boundaries and limitations around these practices. You may hear about something that you couldn't imagine before, an experience that would enrich your own health and well-being. Something you would never have come up with on your own.

It's a lot like a creative community where artists live and work together. They find that their work takes on a new and energized life, with each person lifting up the other and growing together. Some of the work that comes from these intentional communities is the most expansive and beautiful.

We need each other. It's so easy to forget our own ability to heal. We hold ourselves captive in the "I don't know how to do this right" thinking. There is no right way to imagine. Some people can visualize, while others are not visual but can feel what it's like to heal. Yet others may connect to imagery through the other senses. The health-care systems we have right now tell us that healing happens outside of us. We are told that drugs or surgery can heal us, or doctors have the answers we need to heal. This is what keeps us believing that we are not responsible for our own health, but the reality is that much of what heals us are our own beliefs about healing. Moving from an external to an internal locus of control can be unfamiliar and disorienting, but extremely helpful in our own healing process.

I had a neighbor who once asked me what I did for a living. I told her I teach yoga to people with heart disease. When I told her about how we used imagery as one of the healing practices, her eyes lit up. "I know all about that. It saved my life. I don't usually tell people because they might think I'm crazy, but when I was a little girl, my father died. I was only about five years old, and it was a very hard time for my mother. Shortly after that I was diagnosed with leukemia. I knew that my mother couldn't take any more suffering and she needed me to be ok, so at night when I was lying in my bed, I would imagine little fairies coming into my room, and they would come into my body with their wands and start to heal me. I could actually feel it working." She was so young and yet so wise, with a deep connection to her own inner healer. The image was the perfect image for a five-year-old girl. She believed she could heal herself.

Recently, I ran into her husband, and he told me she had passed away at fifty-five from cancer, that it finally got her. I told him that I tell her story often. He told me with tears in his eyes that she would love that. She felt those fifty extra years were a gift.

Once I heard her story, I started to play with that image myself, imagining little light fairies delivering healing energy with their wands. There is something so delightful about that image, even for an adult. When we share our stories of healing, we invite others to benefit from our self-healing. We all need reminding of how powerful we are, and that our body can resolve some of our most difficult issues if we let it. It can also direct us to the most effective healing practices or tools if we ask.

NON-SPECIFIC IMAGERY

Our bodies are always seeking balance and health. When we cut a finger, the body rises up to heal it. We don't have to do anything; the body rallies on its own and does what it can in every circumstance to maintain our health and well-being. Chronic stress can get in the way of the body's natural healing response to pain or illness. There are different kinds of stress, and many are lifestyle related. Things like diet, exercise, and the way we respond to the difficult and challenging situations of our lives are all ways that can inhibit or expand our body's natural healing responses. If we can engage the mind in something uplifting, it has the power to reset the mind and the nervous system.

Research has shown that imagery can even stimulate changes in our bodily functions such as heart rate, blood pressure, and respiratory patterns.[4] When we bring our body and mind into a peaceful and balanced state, healing can occur naturally. Just this gentle nudge of remembering what it felt like when we were feeling radiant, balanced, harmonious, and joy-filled sparks our immune system and healing begins.

When our senses are engaged in beauty, it lifts our spirit out of the ordinary into the extraordinary and profound. We are then free to experience ourselves in more expansive ways. This can shift our consciousness and illuminate our awareness. That is why recalling images of peace through our imagination can be equally healing for the nervous system, mind, and heart. We can tuck these images into our cellular memory and use them to invoke a healing response when needed. This practice is called non-specific imagery, and it allows us to use the mind and senses to heal ourselves.

Non-Specific Imagery Practice

Before you practice, try to recall a place in nature where you felt at peace and deeply connected. It may have been when you were hiking or walking by the ocean or a lake or watching the full glory of a sunset. It may have been in a flower garden or on a mountain trail. As you recall it, try to invoke all your senses. You may even notice a feeling of peace come over you as you remember the details. It's this feeling we will work with in the following exercise.

- Begin by sitting in a chair or lying on the floor.
- Allow yourself to be comfortable and relaxed.

- Gently take your attention inward and allow your breath to become slow and rhythmic.

- Allowing your mind to rest invokes a deep sense of calm and quiet.

- Begin to remember a place in nature that has inspired you to linger in serenity or awe. It could be near a body of water, along a mountain trail, looking out at a sunrise or sunset, at a bonfire, or even a cozy spot under a tree in your own yard.

- Let the image settle in your mind and heart.

- Imagine as many details as you can. What does the air smell like? What sounds are present? How does the air feel on your skin? Is it warm or cool? Is the air wet or dry? What does it look like when you look around you?

- Begin to let the beauty that surrounds you permeate your being.

- Allow your connection to nature to fill you with a sense of peace and serenity.

- Hold onto that feeling as you access a sense of harmony and balance in your whole body.

- Allow that feeling of harmony to awaken a healing response.

- Rest in that for several minutes.

- When you feel ready to come out, make a conscious connection to that feeling of healing, and allow yourself to return to it often.

HOW WE TALK TO OURSELVES AND OTHERS MATTERS

When someone speaks to our heart, we feel it. There is a buoyancy and knowingness that comes from words that touch our hearts. We feel it when someone is trying to lift us up, and we feel it when there is another agenda. We all know people who just make us feel good. They radiate kindness and compassion. Their words fall on us like nourishment. Even people we don't know can have this effect on us.

I recall a sweet experience I had one day at the gym as I trudged up the three flights of stairs to do my usual walk on the treadmill. Nebraska winters almost never encourage a long walk outside, so I resign myself to a few months of indoor walking. On this day I happened to look up, and my eyes caught a young woman who looked right at me and smiled so big that my heart felt like it grew. It was a smile of connection and warmth. She could have walked right past but instead chose a heart connection. This brief feeling of connection stayed with me like a ray of sunshine that inspired me to pass it on.

We all have the power to impact someone else's life by our choice of actions and words, and yet, most of all, we can impact our own lives by the way we act and talk to ourselves. What we tell ourselves also has the undeniable power to lift us up or keep us down. We hear everything we say to ourselves, even when we don't say it out loud. Our internal dialogue is what shapes our experiences with others and the world around us.

One day I was working at a coffee shop with my friend Patrick, and I was feeling my usual frustration with my lack of computer skills. "Sometimes, I'm so stupid!" I blurted out. He looked at me and in a deep and compassionate voice responded, "Don't talk like that about my good friend." His words shook me. I would never talk about someone else like that, so why would I think this was an appropriate way to speak to myself? Somehow, we have gotten the message that we can speak to ourselves in ways that would be considered unacceptable if we spoke that way to others. Why aren't we important enough to treat with simple respect and consideration?

We all know about the plant experiments that show how speaking nicely to plants affects their growth.[5] We are all like plants, just with more complicated emotions. We need to speak to ourselves and others with kindness and love in order to build trust and respect, but most of all to flourish and grow.

When my aunt Nancy was in her late fifties, she was diagnosed with leukemia. She spent many days and weeks in the hospital, and her doctor was very negative about her prognosis. Every time he came into the room, he brought a cloud of darkness with him. His words were so negative that she started calling him "Dr. Doom and Gloom." She realized that if she was going to heal, she needed to be spared from *his* constant belief that she was going to die. She asked her children to shield her from him, and she began watching funny movies and videos. I remember hearing that she was laughing and carrying on like a teenager. As soon as she got free of his negative thinking, she was able to see a path for her own healing. She lived well into her nineties and swears that blocking Dr. Doom and Gloom was responsible for her healing.

One thing I appreciate about integrative and lifestyle medicine is that many of the practitioners understand that their words can serve as medicine. They consider the role they have in their clients/patients' healing outcomes. They choose their words wisely and even allow their words to be a part of the treatment protocols. There is an art and science to using words as medicine. If a doctor is not hopeful about your prognosis, it's hard to maintain hope. For some a diagnosis is a relief and for others a weight that can't be lifted or overcome. Either way, what doctors tell us about our ability to heal, we believe. The medical community recognizes the power this suggestion has, and there is no better example than the research that has emerged around the *p*lacebo effect.

For years, research studies have used placebos, which are an inactive treatment such as sugar pills to try to understand the impact or success of an active drug. The researchers then compare the outcomes of the groups taking the placebo with those of the ones taking the actual drug, to understand the success or failure of the drug. In an article published in *Harvard Magazine*, Cara

Feinberg states that "researchers have found that placebo treatments—interventions with no active drug ingredients—can stimulate real physiological responses, from changes in heart rate and blood pressure to chemical activity in the brain, in cases involving pain, depression, anxiety, fatigue, and even some symptoms of Parkinson's."[6]

In a blog from Harvard Health, Robert H. Shmerling, MD, says, "The power of suggestion is a double-edged sword. If you expect a treatment to help you, it may be more likely to do so. And if you expect a treatment will be harmful, you are more likely to experience negative effects. That phenomenon is called the 'nocebo effect.' For example, if you tell a person that a headache is a common side effect of a particular medication, that person is more likely to report headaches even if they are actually taking a placebo. The power of expectation is formidable and probably plays a significant role in the benefits *and* the side effects of commonly prescribed medications."[7] Just this research alone on the placebo and nocebo effect offers credibility to the world of imagery and the power of self-talk to shape our experience.

IMAGINING A POSITIVE OUTCOME

Imagery can also help us in our everyday lives. We can use it to accomplish goals that make our lives meaningful and productive. Even small tasks can be made easier with imagery. When you think about the last time you accomplished something, you may be able to retrace the thoughts that preceded it. Often, those thoughts include some kind of imagery. Things as simple as cooking, preparing for a meeting at work, meeting an exercise goal, planning a vacation, completing a project, or achieving other health goals can be more effective with the addition of imagery.

I have been an anxious flier for many years. It can make my travels so uncomfortable. At some point I realized that my worry and anxiety was making it worse. I noticed that when I could focus my attention on arriving safely, my mind was resting in a more positive place. Now, each time I fly, I imagine the plane wrapped in white or golden light. I think of the elements and how they support the plane in the air. Sometimes, with a sense of deep gratitude, I say to the wind element, "Oh glorious wind, please give support to this plane as it makes its way with ease and grace to its destination." I may even talk to the earth element and ask for support during takeoff and landing. I will then envision the takeoff, the smooth easy ride through the air, followed by a graceful landing. I will replay this image several times in my mind. Then I remind myself that I have done what I can do from my end. I take a deep sigh and settle into my breath. This simple imagery practice keeps me from looping into the anxiety I feel in my body, slowly replacing the old negative pathways with a new and uplifting message.

INTENTION SETTING

Our lives form around our intentions whether they are conscious or unconscious. When we create an intention that is thoughtful and deliberate, we can begin to change the shape our life takes. If we can see it differently, we can begin to make choices about our actions that lead to an outcome we are hoping for. We forget that our lives are mostly a reflection of all our choices. When we set intentions, we are taking responsibility for those choices, and we are sculpting an outcome of our own choosing. While sometimes we don't have control over things that happen in our lives, we do always have a choice about how we react to what we are given. These choices can then shape future outcomes. Essentially this is the cycle of cause and effect. Ultimately, our thoughts create our intentions, and our intentions have the power to manifest into actions.

When looking to set an intention, it's helpful if it aligns with our higher purpose or what we are meant to be or do in the world. Each one of us has unique gifts or talents to offer the world. When we offer those in the service of others, we feel a sense of purpose that brings us into harmony with our own spirit. Our sense of purpose can be found in what excites us. It tends to be something we are naturally good at, or the things we are drawn to. Often it is right in front of us.

When we tune into our hearts and look to the wisdom of our own hearts to lead us, we can uncover our deeper purpose and align with that. Meditation can help us tune into the depths of our being and listen to our calling. It can clear away the clutter and bring what matters to the foreground.

Another practice is to write down the things you love to do, and then write down the things you are particularly good at. Lastly, write down the things that excite and inspire you. As you observe the things on your lists, notice any patterns. This process can give you insight into your own purpose. As you uncover your purpose, you can use your intentions to support and nurture it.

It's important to realize that stating a positive intention doesn't mean you don't have negative feelings or challenges. It's necessary to let all the ways you are feeling and thinking arise without trying to suppress or push them down. Intentions are a way of turning your focus to what you want to feed, because what you feed grows.

When setting an intention, it is important to imagine it as if you were already living it, as if it were already so. This is why stating your intention in the first person is so helpful. Using "I am" phrases, or phrases that make it personal to you, will direct your intentions with power and purpose.

Here are some examples of intentions:

- My body is healthy and strong.
- I am filled with deep gratitude for my precious life.
- I am connected to my body and respect its needs.
- I take every opportunity to grow and learn from my experiences.

- I am aligned with my own creative force and access it with ease.
- I am open and adventurous.
- I am connected to a higher power and can feel the influence of that power in my life.
- I am grounded and calm.
- I trust that my life is unfolding as it should.
- I am present and aware, and that presence guides me.
- I am filled with compassion for myself and those around me.
- I flow with life's ups and down with ease and grace.
- I prioritize my health and well-being with self-care.
- I trust myself and my intuition.
- I am safe and at peace at this moment.
- I am radiant and full of life.

Our held beliefs about our healing affect our outcomes. When people have given up, the words and tone they use reflect that resignation. And when people believe they will heal and recover, their hope and vision is evident. Those who talk to themselves with encouragement and love will often draw that experience to themselves. Our intentions have a powerful role in our own health outcomes.

It can be helpful to practice intention setting after a practice of deep relaxation or meditation, so the body and mind are centered and relaxed. You can also use the following shortened version.

Intention-Setting Practice
Before you begin, choose something you want more of in your life. Something you would like to feed and give energy to. This

may be something you are already working on or with, or it may be something for just this moment. If you're not sure, feel free to look over the previous intention list and use or modify something on that list.

- Find somewhere to sit or lie down.
- Take a few long, slow, deep breaths and begin to relax.
- Let your body and mind settle.
- Direct your breath into any areas of tension and encourage them to soften.
- Now send a wave of relaxation from top to toe, smoothing out any remaining tension.
- Begin to settle with yourself just as you are.
- Settle with the current conditions of your body and mind.
- Breathe as if your whole body could breathe.
- Begin to call to your awareness something you want to bring more of into your life. Something that aligns with your purpose (what you are meant to be and do in this world).
- Repeat this as if you were speaking it from your heart.
- Say it as if it were already so, as if you were already living it.
- Say it slowly several times.
- Pause and just listen.
- Again say it slowly several times.
- When you are finished, slowly open your eyes, and sit quietly for a few moments before returning to your activities.

Over the next few hours and days, return to this intention and repeat it. Begin to watch as it takes shape in your life. Notice how your actions take shape around your intention, and how your intention begins to find its way into action in your own life.

Imagery has applications in everything we do: preparing for a meeting or a test, making a meal, planning a trip, presenting an idea to a group, competing in a tournament, speaking in front of others, playing sports, preparing for a surgery, when we need to heal, when we need to have a hard conversation, and so much more. In all the situations where we feel stress and anxiety, imagery can help us find our way through with a bit more confidence and ease. The more we do it, the easier it gets and the better we get at it.

If you feel like you can't do something, imagery can help clear a path in your mind until you are ready to do it. It can help you prepare. When students aren't sure they can do a certain yoga movement, I encourage them to imagine it first. If you can't imagine it, then it's best not to try to physically do it until you *can* imagine it. Trust your imagination. Let it help you open pathways in your mind first.

A healing shift starts as a seed in the mind. We water it with our attention and intention, and we begin to feel it taking root. As we shine our light on it over and over, it grows. As the image of healing blooms in our awareness, a powerful shift occurs. This is the power of manifestation. We all have this power to manifest. It may seem like magic . . . and I like to believe it is.

CHAPTER 7

Compassion

Kindness and Empathy

"We are at a landmark moment in Western medicine in which compassion and empathy are being recognized as a complement to material interventions such as pharmaceuticals and surgical procedures. The result is a form of healing that is more effective than when either approach is used alone."
—DR. LARRY DOSSEY, MD[1]

A CENTERING MOMENT

Sending Healing to Others

- Sit comfortably and quietly.
- Let the gaze of your eyes soften or close your eyes.
- Turn your attention inward and notice your breath.
- As you allow your breath to settle down and smooth out, begin to gently weave the breaths together.

- Gently rest your hands over your heart and imagine that your heart is breathing.
- Now imagine someone who is suffering. This can be anyone that you know personally or someone you don't know personally but you feel for their suffering.
- Begin by breathing in the suffering. Take in the suffering with a wish for their freedom from that suffering.
- And now imagine breathing out space, healing, and relief.
- Do this for several breaths. Take in the suffering with a wish for their freedom from that suffering. Breathe out space and healing and relief from suffering.
- Rest your attention for a few moments in the spaces of your own heart.
- Make a slow and gentle transition when you are ready.

THE WOMAN IN THE GROCERY STORE IS IN THE TEN ITEMS OR less lane with fifteen items. I look over her shoulder with a bit of judgment and anger. "Doesn't she know how to read?" I think to myself. Then I hear her explain to the checker in a faint and somber tone, "My father just passed away this morning and I need to get my mom a few things. I'm sorry if I have too many items." At that moment I felt ashamed. I remember when my dad passed away and the feeling of overwhelm in wanting to support my mom in any way I could. I imagine it was all this woman could do, to get herself to the store and pick up a few items, let alone wait in a long checkout line while grieving the loss of her father. I felt compassion rising in my heart, and I wished I could have led with that compassion, knowing full well we are all living with or through something.

The word *compassion* comes from the Latin root *passio*, which means "to suffer," paired with the Latin prefix *com*, meaning "together." To suffer together. It puts us right in the middle of things. When we have compassion, we are "with" someone. People will confuse compassion with sympathy, but the word *sympathy* means having a feeling of pity or sorrow for someone else's misfortune. When we pity, we don't include ourselves in that suffering. It isolates the person suffering and puts us at a distance.

In some ways sympathy is a protective response. We feel sad for someone but hope their suffering won't touch us. How many times have we shied away from a friend whose partner just died, or whose teenager was facing addiction or suffering from an eating disorder? Sometimes avoiding the situation seems easier, but that response will likely affect the relationship in the long run. On the other hand, how often do we make it a priority to connect with someone we know who is suffering, to hold them with compassion and sit alongside them while they are in pain? While it may take effort and energy to make the call or show up for that person, our presence is healing. Additionally, it illustrates our own ability to be present with ourselves and the moment.

Compassion can be learned and practiced through cultivating the ability to feel what it must be like to be in someone else's shoes, to deeply hear and understand someone. What would it be like to have lived another's life, with all the circumstances and conditioning they have had? What must it be like to be them right now with what they are going through? Compassion helps us listen, feel, and care. When we listen in these deep and understanding ways, it's healing for others and ourselves. It creates an openness that breaks down barriers and walls by cultivating kindness and love. It invites us to hold the suffering of others and ourselves, even when we feel scared or on shaky ground. This requires awareness, courage, and practice on our part, but when we have the wisdom and buoyancy to do this, it can be like a life raft for those who need somewhere or something to hold onto.

Not only would we like to feel seen and heard by friends and family, but we also all want to feel seen and heard in the doctor's office. As we discussed in chapter 6, the power of words and held beliefs influence our healing. We need medical doctors to believe us when we tell them about our suffering, we need them to respond compassionately and with empathy, and we need them to believe in our healing. Unfortunately, there is research that shows that empathy in medical staff can decrease across the years of medical school, highlighting the importance of teaching empathy and compassion as necessary skills to medical students. Empathy and compassion are critical skills for medical doctors because "a growing body of research has established the importance of empathy in several key aspects of medicine. Physician empathy leads to improved patient satisfaction, greater adherence to therapy, better clinical outcomes, and lower malpractice liability."[2] Fortunately, there are places like Stanford Medicine's Center for Compassion and Altruism Research and Education where they are pursuing research addressing teaching compassion in community and health-care settings.[3] These projects and the emerging data suggest that there is something worth investigating in the world of medicine that may not be as tangible as drugs or surgery.

However, it doesn't take research to know that when we feel heard and understood, something almost magical happens. It invokes a healing response. We find ourselves lifted up and supported. We feel connected to others who see us, and that connection, in and of itself, is healing.

We all have come face-to-face with the suffering of others. The news is filled with people having to flee their homes and seek shelter somewhere else during wildfires, tornadoes, hurricanes, and even war. When someone loses a child or a loved one, this brings us into direct contact with our own feelings of fear, loss, and sadness. And although we may not want to admit it, after the initial sadness, we might experience other feelings such as relief: "I'm so glad it wasn't me or my family." Our discomfort with suffering urges us to exit our feelings of compassion and take a sigh of relief that it wasn't us. This feeling illustrates how hard it is to really sit in someone else's suffering for more than a couple of minutes.

How can we open our hearts and stay present with the suffering of others without being overcome by it? When we feel pity "for" someone, we are disconnected. We are responding from a place that allows us to stay separate from another person's experience. Feeling "with" someone invites us into the shared feelings of another.

Compassion arises naturally when we feel ourselves in alignment "with" the other person. When we sharpen our ability to stay with someone else's experience and really soak in what it must feel like to be in their life, something extraordinary emerges. We let down our guard and join another person's reality. We feel a connection.

In order to hold space for another, we must first be willing to rest in our own suffering and discomfort. This takes practice and patience. Meditation can be an excellent tool to help teach us this skill, since meditation is the practice of learning to sit with ourselves. It teaches us to be mindful in each moment and to observe the ways we try to exit. It helps us stay in the present moment. When thoughts and feelings arise, we stay still and observe our own reactions and feelings without judging or labeling. We let ourselves witness without getting lost in the storyline. We keep returning to the moment over and over again. Over time we train our minds and hearts to be still and open to whatever arises. This way we build our sense of tolerance. It is tolerance that fuels compassion. When we practice tolerance, especially in the most challenging moments, it leads to compassion, and ultimately, compassion leads us to love. It is love that heals us. It heals our hearts, and it heals our communities. As Martin Luther King Jr. said, "Love is the only force capable of turning an enemy into a friend."[4]

In my work as a stress management specialist, I have been witness to the gathering of groups with diverse backgrounds. At first I wonder how they will tolerate each other given the differences in their age, culture, ethnicity, socioeconomic background, gender identities, and held beliefs. With just a few common goals and an environment of respect guided by compassionate listening, it was heartwarming to watch what in other circumstances might be a highly volatile situation turn into a landscape of tolerance, compassion, and community. If someone would have told me that a self-proclaimed anti-gay activist would be lovingly sitting at the bedside of a gay man who was nursing his partner in the last days of life, I would never have believed it. Yet this is what happens when we open our hearts and find our shared humanity. Appreciating our differences and the diversity of ideas and thoughts helps us expand our own consciousness and experience.

If we really want to have a centered heart, it requires letting go of the feelings of separation that lead us to believe we are somehow not on the same team. When we remember that humanity is our shared team, we work together and not against each other. Nothing illustrates this more than when there is a disaster. People of all faiths, cultures, colors, and genders come together to support and help each other.

As a citizen of Ukraine, my dear friend Daria has been living through the painful reality of the war in her country. When she tells her story, in the midst of the horror is a light that shines from the hearts of people coming together to support and care about each other. She describes the ravages of the land and cultural centers, the power outages, the air raids, and the limited supplies. The hardship is palpable, yet tucked in those stories are the stories of humanity, courage, and love—the people in the air raid shelters coming together and supporting each other, the elderly woman shop owner in the darkness helping Daria find the right shade of lipstick and the right piece of clothing so she could feel some sense of normalcy in all the loss and chaos. The stories of friends and family coming together to help and support each other are the stories that rise to the top. They are like gems of inspiration and hope. In these moments of hardship, we are called to be the highest version of ourselves. It's as if that resilience and love has always been there, just waiting for a reason to surface.

As a small child, I remember my father talking about the Great Depression of 1929. As he would tell his story of adversity, I could feel his longing for a bygone time. A time when people came together to help each other. The differences in their beliefs or ethnicity didn't matter; they were part of something bigger. During that time, his mother, my grandmother, made food for those who had nothing to eat, and would offer it in return for anyone who wanted to work in her garden. She didn't really care about the work, but she wanted them to feel pride and dignity. She didn't ask if they held the same beliefs or values as she did. She didn't care about their religion. They were suffering and she felt it was her responsibility to help in whatever way she could.

During the COVID-19 pandemic, there were so many stories of people coming together to help others, yet there was another story that emerged at the same time. Aside from the devastating effects of COVID-19 and the isolation from friends and family, there was also a division that permeated our lives. We were constantly confronted with choosing sides. While we were fighting about which treatment or health behavior was the "best" or most scientific, we were stepping further and further away from each other and our own humanity. Was it the media that kept us captive in this "us or them" rhetoric? Or was it just the pull of fear on our fragile lives that had us putting our fists up? "Are you with us or against us?" was the powerful and resounding anthem. The stance of "fists up" creates stress in our bodies and minds. It triggers our sympathetic nervous system, known as our fight or flight response, and it closes the pathway of communication and love. It is the opposite position of compassion. Compassion has us put down our fists and open our hearts to each other. There is clearly a time and place to fight for what we believe in, but maintaining our humanity and respect for each other can always be a priority.

The more we lock ourselves away from others, the more fear and anger we can use to rally against someone. Have you ever noticed how much easier it is to be angry with someone when you are driving in a car, or talking on the phone, or worse yet, posting on social media? We are much more likely to lash out when we aren't face-to-face with the person we are interacting with. When we start to dehumanize others and separate ourselves from them, it opens the door to being able to hurt another person.

I used to find myself muttering under my breath at other drivers. At some point that muttering became full-on grumbling and swearing. I admit, when it happens, it is not my proudest moment. One afternoon I was driving with my friend Tony, who caught me in the act of my uncensored grumbling. He said to me with such tenderness, "Oh Susi, you don't know what he might be going through. Maybe he's trying to get to the hospital to see his dying grandmother. Maybe he just lost his job. Maybe he was just diagnosed with a terrible illness." Giving someone the benefit of the doubt is what we would want if the tables were turned. This requires seeing someone's humanity.

Now, my practice is to look at the other drivers or people in the cars around me and try to imagine what they must be dealing with in their lives right now. This has helped my driving behavior immensely, and I save myself the wear and tear on my own nervous system when I don't get lost in the negative emotions that arise when another driver cuts me off. I am also able to recognize that the irritation I have for the other drivers is more about myself than them. I am responsible for my reactions and my own experience. Reframing how I want to see and experience my external circumstances is my superpower.

When we cultivate compassion, the mind is not caught up in feelings of anger, resentment, bitterness, or jealousy. The mind can rest, and we stop reacting in ways that leave us feeling stressed and overwhelmed. We are less likely to see ourselves as separate from someone else, and we begin to see and live the shared human experience.

In the tradition of Yoga, there are ten ethical principles called Yamas and Niyamas, which serve as a foundation for living in harmony with ourselves and others. These precepts help us align with our best selves. They serve to loosen those attachments that keep us caught in a cycle of negative thinking and negative emotions. When we can release those attachments, the mind is free to experience the positive impact of meditation and love. The very first and most important of these guiding principles is called Ahimsa, which translates to non-violence or non-harming. While non-harming may sound simple, it is quite nuanced. It calls us to observe our thoughts, words, and deeds with attention and care. Inherent in these precepts are the positive actions we can take to bring these principles into our lives.

The instruction for practicing Ahimsa is the cultivation of kindness, compassion, and respect for all beings. As we direct our attention to our own actions, we begin to notice how our choices about our treatment of ourselves and others has a powerful impact on what we attract into our lives. If we treat others with kindness, we invite kindness into our own lives. If we approach others with aggression and anger, we also bring those qualities to our lives. The escalation of violence or the escalation of peace is a choice. Not only does Ahimsa ask us to regard other people with compassion and respect, but it also asks us to treat *all* beings with this same kindness, including animals. Animals share with humans the same emotions of fear, anxiety, joy, and stress. Their nervous systems experience stress much like what ours do. They, too, are sentient beings. Our disregard for their lives is a disregard for the diversity that is crucial to our survival on this earth. When we give up eating animals, not only do we promote the health of our physical heart,[5] but there is healing on an emotional level that comes from not imposing harm on another living being.

For some, the decision to go to a plant-based diet comes from a desire to enlist healthier lifestyle choices; for others it is a response to the harm inflicted on animals. When my friend was just six years old, she witnessed a Kosher slaughtering. That moment caused her to give up eating meat for her entire life. She was so affected by this experience that it changed her relationship to animals as food forever. She couldn't imagine sacrificing an animal's life so she could have one meal.

There is a very vivid description in Melanie Joy's book *Why We Love Dogs, Eat Pigs, and Wear Cows* that brings awareness to our choices around the consumption of animals.[6] She outlines a dinner party where the host is serving a delicious stew. When asked for the recipe, the host, without missing a beat, replies, "You begin with five pounds of golden retriever meat, well-marinated." None of us would ever consider serving a golden retriever stew for dinner, yet we are somehow okay with serving cows and pigs and chickens. Ahimsa asks us to consider our actions and make choices that help us align with a more compassionate lifestyle. Becoming a vegetarian or vegan is not only a compassionate practice toward animals, but also exhibits compassion for the planet since factory farms are causing major concerns with climate change.[7] Not only that, but it is also a loving practice for our own physical health and emotional well-being. The research on low-fat vegan and plant-based diets is mounting as a pathway to living a longer, healthier life.[8] In my work with Ornish Lifestyle Medicine, our team taught five lifestyle practices, outlined by Dr. Ornish, to stop and reverse heart disease.[9] A low-fat, plant-based diet, moderate daily exercise, group support, and the stress management practices described in his book *Undo It!* are at the core of his life-changing research and decades-long work.[10]

Not only is it helpful to explore our relationship to animals as food but also our relationships to animals as pets. How do we treat our pets? There is mounting research on the positive impact that pets have on our cardiovascular and mental health.[11] When we care for another being, we open our hearts to giving and receiving love. In the year 2022, 70 percent of US households, or about 90.5 million families, owned a pet. Pet ownership not only expands our own capacity for compassion, but it seems that animals are in turn showing us compassion. In 2011, the National Service Animal Registry had 2,400 service and emotional support animals in its registry; in 2022, there were nearly 200,000.[12] It seems that we need the love of our pets as much or more than they need our love.

When I traveled to India years ago, I was struck by the way so many animals roamed the streets. At one point, on the streets of Delhi, I noticed an elephant walking behind me. It was decorated in brightly colored chalk with a slight, young man riding on its back. No one seemed at all surprised, except me. Growing up in the United States, I was taught to fear animals that aren't in cages, but in India the cows, elephants, donkeys, monkeys, and even the occasional pig seemed to share the streets with people. I felt the deep sense of connection and respect that people had toward the animal kingdom there. It offered me a different way to think about my relationship to nature and animals. When we live in harmony with animals and nature, it can reduce feelings of loneliness and decrease levels of cortisol, the stress hormone, in the blood.[13] It can lower blood pressure and increase feelings of social support. Simply put, we just feel healthier and happier when we live in harmony with all beings.

Self-Compassion

For many of us, having compassion for animals or others feels more natural than extending compassion to ourselves, yet self-compassion provides the foundation for how we treat others. When we feel happy and in balance, compassion arises in us almost effortlessly. When we feel good, we want the best for others. As a yoga therapist, I hear the perfectionism, shame, judgment, self-loathing, and guilt that others inflict upon themselves.

It's heartbreaking to hear how hard we can be on ourselves. This can get played out in our relationships with others in the form of projection as well.

What we don't like about others is often a reflection of something that we struggle with or are unwilling to see in our own self. This may be a hard pill to swallow, but if you think about a relationship that you struggle with, often there is some aspect of yourself that you are reacting to. At the very least, there is some learning available in our relational struggles. When we have a powerful reaction to someone, it is usually a signal that there is something there for us to look into, for better or for worse.

The good news is that what we love about others can also be a reflection of the qualities we possess ourselves. When I train yoga teachers, we end our nine months of study with a graduation ceremony. It's a time for teachers to reflect on their own value and what they have to offer others. My friend and colleague Patrick used to lead the session with a very powerful exercise taken from the work of Maria Nemeth, author of *Mastering Life's Energies*.[14]

I offer it here as a practice.

Make sure to go step by step without reading ahead. Grab a notebook or paper and pencil to begin.

- Think about someone you admire, someone you look up to.

- Now think about the qualities you respect, love, or appreciate in that person.

- Write them down. You can write as much as you like (e.g., you might think of your grandma and write things like "loving," "gentle," "kind," "sensitive," "a great cook," "a jokester," and "witty").

- Now do it with two more people you admire.

- As you read through the qualities, you might see duplicates. That's fine, just cross out the duplicates and keep going.

- Now use a clean sheet to write down all the qualities you have compiled.

- Next, put the words "I am" in front of each quality.

- At the end of your list write, "I know these are mine because I see them in others."

- Now, read out loud each "I am" quality you have written about those you admire. For example, "I am loving," "I am kind," "I am sensitive," and so on.

- Complete the list with the sentence, "I know these are mine because I see them in others."

- It is important to pay attention as you hear yourself recite the beautiful qualities you see in others, realizing that these are also qualities *you* possess.

Having this list of qualities that you embody helps you regard yourself with the same respect and admiration that you hold for others. This self-love sets the ground for your own well-being and happiness. As we apply self-love and compassion to our interactions, we begin to see that our happiness comes from our own reactions and responses to what is happening around us and within us. How do we shift our reactions? The ancient Yoga Sutras of Patanjali offer suggestions for maintaining our peace of mind by using the four keys for unlocking happiness cited in sutra 1:33.[15] Through the understanding and practice of each, we can begin to manage our everyday responses to what is happening around us.

THE FOUR KEYS FOR UNLOCKING HAPPINESS
1. Friendliness Toward the Happy
We can all remember those feelings we had as children when someone else received something that we wanted but didn't have. This feeling of jealousy can keep us from experiencing our own happiness. If we go through our lives always wanting what others

have, we will never find our own happiness. We also end up missing the important and meaningful moments in others' lives. If we cultivate feelings of friendliness when someone is happy, it allows us to avoid getting lost in jealousy or bitterness. By cultivating friendliness toward those who are happy, we also experience happiness, and this protects our inner sense of calm.

2. Compassion for the Unhappy

For many of us, our instinct may be to shield ourselves from those who are unhappy or to secretly rejoice in the fact that it isn't us that has to endure their discomfort. But shielding or secret pleasure, which is a normal human defense, also keeps us from sharing deep and meaningful relationships with those around us. Being able to sit with someone and feel a sense of compassion teaches us how to feel for others. It also teaches us how to sit with our own discomfort and have compassion for ourselves in difficult times.

3. Delight and Joy for the Virtuous

When someone is committed to high ethical and moral values, we say they are virtuous. When they act in a virtuous way, it can leave us feeling "less" honorable or in competition with their actions. Envy keeps us from appreciating the virtues of others. Feeling delight for the virtuous is another way to protect our inner peace. When we can find a sense of joy when we see others acting in honorable and noble ways, we feed our own nobility and integrity. This helps us remain balanced and inspired.

4. Disregard for the Non-Virtuous

In some ways, this may be the most difficult key to unlock. When people are acting in ways that seem unethical or even egregious, we feel the need to fight back or do something that draws even more attention to their behavior. Yoga teaches us to disregard and even turn our attention completely away from these kinds of behaviors. By engaging in battle, we give energy to these situations and cause them to get bigger. We all know too well that anger and violence breed more anger and more violence. This has been the stance of so many of our great and powerful leaders like Martin Luther King Jr., Gandhi, and the Dalai Lama. When we turn away and don't give energy to these kinds of behaviors, we stop feeding them. They then lose their power over us, and we stop giving away the power to control our happiness to someone else.

LISTENING WITH COMPASSION

Learning to listen with compassion is a skill that brings us closer to others. It breaks down walls and lets us feel connection and love. When I worked with participants in Ornish Lifestyle Medicine, I was able to witness firsthand the importance of compassionate listening in the group support element of the program. The group was a place for participants to practice their communication skills as well as practice the vulnerability of sharing feelings with others. The camaraderie and respect that was nurtured gave rise to a deep sense of community, love, and healing. One thread that runs through compassionate listening is the belief that others have their own answers and the capacity to handle what life is offering them no matter what.

Below are some suggestions and guidelines for listening with compassion:

No Judgment

We can all get caught up in passing judgment from time to time, and not judging does require some restraint. It's important to watch not only what we say, but what we think. When we judge someone, we shut the door on staying open to what they are feeling. It stops the flow of compassion and love.

No Advice

Giving advice tells the other person that we think they need something from us, and it can make them feel that we don't think they are capable of finding their own answers. To have faith in someone's ability to find their own solutions is a gift we can give someone that will help strengthen their own inner resources.

No Problem Solving

Again, when we try to solve problems for others, it tells them we are not confident in their own ability to find solutions. It also takes us away from the feelings they are expressing and doesn't allow them to be heard and held. It's like skipping over the most important part of the story to get to the ending.

No Reassurance

It's hard to resist offering reassurance to someone who is suffering. In some ways this may be one of the hardest skills to refine. Most of us can shift our judgments and refrain from advice giving or problem solving, but we are like a boat lost at sea if we can't reassure someone that they will be okay when they are deep in it. The truth is, we don't know how it's going to turn out for anyone. Sitting in life's mysteries requires us to let go of wanting to control the outcomes. Sometimes I will say to my husband, "Just tell me it's all going to be okay, even if you aren't sure." He will lovingly do this for me, but in the moments that follow, he will compassionately add, "No matter how it turns out, honey, I'm here for you." Reassuring someone that you will be there for them is quite different from reassuring them that whatever it is they are facing will turn out okay.

No Testimonials

When someone is telling us their story and they feel hopeless, sad, or even beat down, it can be hard to be still and listen. It feels hard to watch someone suffer. We think that if we somehow tell them how it worked for us to find a way out of suffering, it will work for them. We think our story might have value for them. The drawback is that when we launch into our story, we take the focus away from them and put it on us. We let them know that we can't bear their suffering, and our inspiring tale could somehow make it better. We risk our connection when we do this. They have entrusted us with their story, and our biggest gift to them is to listen and respond with empathy and compassion. Instead of launching into your own story, try responding in a way that forms connection, such as, "Gee, I can hear how hard that is for you," "Thank you for sharing your story with me, I appreciate hearing your feelings," "When you talk about your struggles with your father, I feel so connected to you since I share some similar struggles with my own father; tell me more."

When we listen with compassion, we are not trying to fix anything. We are allowing ourselves to be touched by the experience of someone else, and we aren't trying to change or alter what they are feeling or expressing. We are simply holding space for their story to emerge while holding that story with humility and respect.

SPEAKING WITH COMPASSION

Have you ever listened to someone whose words are like medicine? Words have power. They have the power to hurt, harm, help, or heal. In the ancient Sufi tradition, they say that speech should pass through the following three gates before leaving your lips: Is it true, is it kind, is it necessary?

Is It True?

When we speak the truth, we invite truthfulness into our lives. Have you ever been caught in a lie? The amount of energy it takes to manage a lie can be exhausting. We tell lies for different reasons. Sometimes we just want to be liked. Other times we think someone else can't handle the truth, so we withhold it. What would happen if we had the courage to speak the truth? If we knew we were "enough" just as we are, and we didn't feel we had to lie so people would like us. What if we had the confidence in others' resilience and ability to hear the truth? How would our lives change? While the truth for one person may not be the truth for someone else, one thing we can aspire to is the bravery to speak our own truth.

Is It Kind?

Refining our words so they reflect a higher level of kindness helps us find more peace in our relationships. Sometimes when we speak what we think is the truth, it can sound unkind or even mean-spirited. Often anger needs to be expressed and not suppressed, but when we take responsibility for our own rage by not projecting onto others, we not only calm down our communication but give permission to others to do the same. It can also be helpful to use "I feel" phrases when letting others know about your feelings—phrases like "I feel angry and disappointed" rather than "I'm angry at you" or "you are a disappointment." This keeps the inflammation down and allows the other person to be more receptive. They aren't being blamed or shamed. It leaves room for them to be curious and open.

Is It Necessary?

Some of the words we speak aren't necessary. Idle gossip or slander are never necessary. In the moment, it may feel like a release of our pent-up energy or like we are bonding with someone when we talk badly about someone else, but in the end, it only lets that person know that you may speak badly about them, too. It breaks the trust we are ultimately looking for in our relationships. However, talking with respect about how we feel to someone can deepen our trust and friendship.

In the tradition of yoga, practicing silence has been a helpful tool for understanding the power of speech. It can help us preserve our energy and become more thoughtful with our words. Doing a silent retreat or just taking a day to be in silence can point to the ways we use our voice and our energy. Practicing silence informs our speech and the importance of our words.

COMPASSION PRACTICES
Meditation to Inspire Compassion
You can record your voice reading this practice (and the following one) on your phone or computer so you can practice whenever you want. Or visit www.yourcenteredheart.com for guided audio practices.

- Sit up or lie down in a comfortable position.
- Gently close your eyes.
- Allow your attention to move inward.
- Begin to direct your attention to the breath.
- Gently follow the breath as it comes in and as it goes out.
- Scan your body for any held tension, and send your breath to those areas as you begin to soften them.
- Now let your awareness rest in your heart center.
- Begin to breathe as if your own heart were breathing in, as if your own heart were breathing out (it may be helpful to place your hand or hands over your heart).
- Let your awareness rest on the breath in your heart.
- If your mind wanders, gently return to the breath in your own heart.
- Sit quietly for several moments.
- Now imagine your own heart connected to everyone breathing and living.
- Imagine all hearts connected and breathing as one heart.
- Feel the sense of connection to others as you send out feelings of understanding compassion in the form of light or energy.

The Practice of Cultivating Compassion

- Lie down in a comfortable position.

- Let your body settle and relax.

- Imagine your whole body breathing in and your whole body breathing out.

- Begin to imagine someone you love; hold them in your heart and imagine what it must be like to be in their life and to live in their circumstances.

- Begin to send them understanding, compassion, and love. Hold them in your heart for several breaths and let their image and that feeling of compassion for them dissolve into your heart.

- Now repeat this practice with someone you are neutral about, a person you may not have strong feelings for either way.

- Bring their image into your heart and hold it there as you try to imagine what it might be like to have lived their life with all their conditioning and circumstances.

- Send them compassion and understanding. Hold their image in your heart for several breaths.

- Now let their image and that feeling of compassion dissolve into your heart.

- Now repeat this with someone you have a small conflict with, someone you normally feel is a friend or you appreciate them, but you may have things that you differ on. Perhaps you have even argued about something recently.

- Bring their image into your heart and hold it there as you try to imagine what it might be like to have lived their life with all their conditioning and circumstances.

- Send them compassion and understanding. Hold their image in your heart for several breaths.

- Now let their image and those feelings of compassion and understanding dissolve into your heart.
- Lastly, repeat this with yourself, holding your own image in your heart. Go through these steps with yourself.
- Send understanding and compassion to yourself, and then let the image dissolve into your heart along with the feelings of understanding and compassion.
- Let yourself linger in these feelings for yourself before coming out of the practice.
- Breathe as if your heart were breathing. Rest in the spaciousness of your own heart.

In time you can add people to this exercise who are more challenging for you. This will help you build tolerance, compassion, and love. This practice can pave the way to mending your relationships while healing your own heart and community.

Remember that there are times we may find ourselves going over the edge from compassion to identifying with the suffering of another until we feel burned out. There is wisdom and emotional intelligence that we need to develop while we work with compassion. This requires a moment-by-moment awareness of our own capacity to be "in it" with someone else. When we feel overwhelmed or over-identified with another, it may be time to recalibrate. It's important to take some time to practice self-compassion and self-care before returning to the situation. Using the practices in this book to come back to yourself and regain your own energies will help you find balance.

The more we work with the practice of compassion, the more we find our own nervous systems becoming stronger and more resilient. Our stress response begins to shift as we incorporate a broader and more respectful view of the circumstances that have such a powerful influence on our behaviors. When we bring love, respect, and kindness to our interactions, our nervous system starts to settle down and our hearts can open to others. In turn, others' hearts can open to us.

CHAPTER 8

Oneness

Nature Consciousness

"Nature has the power to heal because it is where we are from, it is where we belong, and it belongs to us as an essential part of our health and our survival."

—NOOSHIN RAZANI, MD[1]

A CENTERING MOMENT

Nature Heals

- Begin by sitting or lying down in a comfortable position outside in the elements.

- Make sure you are warm enough, especially if you are doing this in a colder climate.

- For a moment, look around you in every direction. Take a few breaths and look up toward the sky. Keep breathing as you look to your right and then to your left. Now look down at the ground, as you continue to mindfully take in your surroundings.

- Begin to take several conscious, slow, deep breaths.
- Close your eyes or soften your gaze.
- Feel yourself taking in the energy of nature each time you inhale, and settle with that energy as you exhale.
- Notice the parts of your body that are in direct contact with the earth. If sitting in a chair, it may be your feet. Wherever there is a connection, begin to breathe yourself deeper into that connection, as if to sink into the feeling of the earth beneath you. Sink into the pull of gravity.
- Now begin to notice any sounds of nature. Maybe you hear birds chirping or the sound of wind rustling. Let your attention be with the sounds or the silence for just a few moments.
- Next, allow yourself to become aware of any smells in the air. Breathe deeply and take in the scents around you for just a few moments longer.
- Now start to notice the feeling of the wind and/or sun against your skin. Notice the sensations.
- Begin to send a wave of gratitude over your body from top to toe. Gratitude for this precious connection of your body to nature. Gratitude for this precious life.
- Allow yourself to rest in this gratitude for just a few more moments.
- Raise your gaze slowly, and take the time to leisurely transition from this practice.

SINCE THE BEGINNING OF TIME, OUR ANCESTORS HAVE LIVED A life close to nature. They have lived in harmony with nature's rhythms, turned to nature's plants and animals for healing, and consulted with the elements for advice and direction. As our lives have migrated indoors, our connection to Mother Nature has suffered. Instead of walking outside on the earth, we have turned to the treadmill and StairMaster for our exercise, using computer-generated images of nature to simulate being outside when we work out. Instead of eating fresh foods that we have grown or cooked for ourselves, we eat prepared foods and frequent the fast-food drive-thru. Rather than consulting the stars for their infinite wisdom, we go to social media to look for answers. How did we get here, and how do we find our way back?

Our desire to "make life easier" has created a different kind of hardship. We have become more and more stressed and less and less able to cope with the life we have constructed. The more we disconnect from nature, the more disconnected we become from ourselves. We've lost our center. This shift has had dire consequences to our health and to our life on this planet. How do we repair this connection without losing the advances we have worked so hard to achieve?

Some of those answers may be found in the ancient tradition of Ayurveda, a holistic system that allows us to gain and maintain optimal health by living in accordance with the elements of the earth. It offers guidance to help us find balance and heal our relationship to nature, while living in the world in a more harmonious way. Ayurvedic medicine is believed to be over 5,000 years old and is the sister science to yoga. *Ayuh* means "life" and *veda* means "science or wisdom." It is a life science that is rooted in wisdom offering lifestyle practices and interventions that bring balance to the body, mind, spirit, and the environment.

One of the fundamental principles of Ayurveda is Pancha Maha Bhutas, also known as the "Five Great Elements," which recognizes that everything living is part of the five elements of nature. As living beings ourselves, Ayurveda suggests that we are so intimately connected to nature that it lives inside of us in the form of earth, water, fire, air, and space. When we are born, these elements arrange themselves in various patterns to create our own unique "doshas." Your constitution is the inherent balance of three doshas when you are born.

Part of the Ayurvedic approach is to give responsibility to the patient by helping them understand their own particular constitution. By understanding the doshas and the elements contained in each dosha, you create a template for understanding how these elements affect you and your own health. They help us make better choices about our foods, activities, sleep, and self-care.

THE DOSHAS

The three doshas are Vata, Pitta, and Kapha. The Vata dosha is composed of air and space (ether), Pitta is made up of fire and water, and Kapha earth and water. We each embody all three doshas, but one is usually dominant. It is common to pair the doshas with the most dominant first and then the second most dominant next. For example: Vata-Pitta, Pitta-Kapha, Vata-Kapha, and so on.

It's helpful to think about the elements contained in each dosha and the qualities they have in nature. This will give you insight as to how they might express in a similar way within your own body. As we explore each one, you may notice characteristics that feel familiar to you. This may be because it is a more predominant dosha for you. In order to identify your own specific dosha, you can look at several types of characteristics. Below is a brief dosha quiz that might help you discover your primary and secondary dosha, which combined creates your individual constitution.

Completing the dosha quiz: Place a check mark in the column that best describes you. Feel free to choose more than one if one or more equally describe you. Be sure to make your selection based on what has been most true across the majority of your life, rather than your current state or what you strive for. Try to proceed without judgment or justification. Add up all the check marks at the bottom of the quiz.

Body Frame	Thin, petite		Medium		Large, thick	
Body Weight	Trouble gaining		Can gain, but lose quickly		Hard to lose, tendency to gain	
Skin Type	Thin, dry		Smooth, combination skin		Thick, oily	
Hair	Dry, brittle, scarce		Straight, oily, hair loss		Thick, curly, wavy	
Teeth	Big, roomy, thin gums		Medium size, tender gums		Healthy, white, strong gums	
Nose	Uneven shape		Long, pointed		Short, round	
Nails	Dry, rough, thin		Sharp, flexible, long		Thick, smooth, shiny	
Appetite	Irregular		Strong, cannot skip meals		Steady, regular	
Digestion	Irregular		Quick		Slow	
Elimination	Dry, constipation		Loose, diarrhea		Thick, incomplete	
Body Temperature	Often cold		Intolerant of heat		Uncomfortable in cold/damp	
Physical Health Issues	Moving pains		Stomach issues		Respiratory issues	
Mental Health Issues	Tendency for anxiety		Tendency for "burnout" or anger issues		Tendency for depression	
Physical Activity	Always active		Moderate		Slow, measured	
Mental Activity	Always active		Moderate		Calm	
Personality	Talkative, social, outgoing		Purpose-driven action, likes control		Reserved	

(*continued*)

Intellect	Quick, not detailed		Accurate, timely		Paced, exact	
Speech Pattern	Rapid, tangential		Precise, articulate		Slow, monotonous	
Sleep Pattern	Short, broken up		Moderate, sound		Deep, long	
Financial Pattern	Impulsive		Indulgent		Controlled	
Career	Creative arts		Science, engineering		Human relations, caregiving	
TOTALS	VATA		PITTA		KAPHA	

Remember that we have aspects of all of these doshas in each of us, but you will likely lean predominantly toward one or two. Once you find your primary and secondary dosha, it is helpful to learn about each one, as you will find yourself moving in and out of balance with all three.

Vata Dosha

This dosha contains the elements of air and ether (space). Vata constitutions tend to be dry, cold, quick, light, erratic, and change-able (just like the wind or air element). Physical characteristics of a primary Vata Dosha include:

- Tendency to be either very short or very tall
- Irregular features
- Thin and petite
- Pains that move and change

Qualities of a primary Vata Dosha include:

- Restless, prone to anxiety
- Multitasking
- Easily irritated but quick to forgive

- Fast talking, fast walking
- Trouble sleeping
- Erratic eating patterns
- Inconsistent, impulsive
- Expressive, with a tendency to ramble
- Spiritual

A person with a predominant Vata Dosha may walk lightly and quickly. They are often blown like the wind from one thing to the next. They usually have many projects going at once, which makes them feel happy and alive, albeit they may get so lost in those projects they forget to eat and sleep. They talk fast and may jump from topic to topic quickly, sometimes making it hard for others to keep up. They are often forgetful and may lose their keys or purse or any number of things on a daily basis. They have pains that come and go, and can often look like they are having a hard time holding it together, but they seem to do ok and even thrive if you just give them a hug. They are sensitive to both noise and wind, and feel best wearing a hat and bundling up. Vatas love to travel and enjoy meeting new people. They are good listeners and love the connection that conversation and community provide. They make compassionate friends and forgive their enemies quickly. They can be very impulsive and often spend money freely as well. They do best with a regular schedule of sleep and meals and practices that help them feel grounded.

When *in balance* Vatas are joyful, spacious, witty, creative, compassionate, and full of energy. They make good therapists, artists, teachers, and friends. When *out of balance* Vatas can be anxious, unfocused, fearful, and overwhelmed.

A person with a predominant Vata Dosha may experience health issues such as joint pain, anxiety, constipation or diarrhea, dry skin, disturbed sleep, and exhaustion. Vata affects the colon, legs, low back, joints, nervous system, and ears.

Pitta Dosha

This dosha contains the elements of fire and water. Pitta constitutions tend to be oily, hot, assertive, sharp, acidic, and intense. Physical characteristics of a primary Pitta Dosha include:

- Medium body frame
- Balanced proportions
- Sharp features
- Pinkish or yellowish hue to the skin (sometimes freckles)
- Early to gray, with balding in men
- Intolerant of heat

Qualities of a primary Pitta Dosha include:

- Organized and goal-oriented
- Fiery
- Generous
- Controlling
- Bright
- Intelligent
- Charismatic
- Big appetites (food, sex, information)

A person with a predominant Pitta Dosha tends to be very charismatic—you may find yourself instantly attracted to them. They are often the life of the party, telling stories and captivating their listeners.

They are visionaries who are hardworking and know how to take charge. They take on projects and know how to get others motivated to fulfill their vision. They can be intense and may push very hard at work and even suffer from burnout. They are voracious learners. Often, they can't get enough, and can get lost in consuming books, information, food, and even people. They are very generous, and they can make life exciting and fun. If they miss a meal, watch out, that makes them pretty grumpy.

When *in balance* Pittas are giving, energetic, charismatic, astute, and happy. They make good leaders, business owners, speakers, teachers, and actors. When *out of balance*, Pittas can be controlling, judgmental, sarcastic, and even cutting with their words, leaving a field of wounded around them.

A person with a predominant Pitta Dosha may experience health issues such as stomach acid and ulcers, diarrhea, headaches, fevers, skin rashes, burnout, pain, and inflammation. Pitta affects the stomach, intestines, mind, eyes, skin, and emotions.

Kapha Dosha

This dosha contains the elements of water and earth. Kapha constitutions tend to be heavy, slow, cool, oily, fluid, soft, and smooth. Physical characteristics of a primary Kapha Dosha include:

- Sturdy, heavy, or compact body frame
- Strong, wavy, and thick hair
- Bright and soft skin
- Moves slowly
- Resistant to illness

Qualities of a primary Kapha Dosha include:

- Caring, compassionate
- Centered, grounded, patient, reliable
- Slow to learn, but doesn't forget
- Good long-term memory, will hold a grudge
- Possessive

- Prone to depression
- Steady, good endurance
- Loving, nurturing, generous heart

A person who is predominantly Kapha is quite fond of children and pets. You may find them feeding the neighborhood stray animals. They will often take in children or anyone who needs nurturing and love. If you go to their home, you might notice their collections, since it's hard for them to let go of anything due to their deep appreciation for things. They attach to both people and things with depth and loyalty. They are solid and kind, but if you cross them, you may never be able to get in their good graces again. They can be stubborn and immovable once they have made up their mind about something or someone. They are sturdy and hearty but can get stuck easily. They are of course made up of water and earth and together that makes mud, making feeling stuck a keynote for Kaphas. They are sensual and love food, but their digestion is often slow or even sluggish.

You may often catch them yawning and dragging without their coffee or morning pick-me-up. They are not easily rattled but sensitive nonetheless. They move with grace and ease and seem happy in their bodies. As friends they are solid, loyal, and nurturing. They tend to make everyone feel at home with their comforting personalities. They are often referred to as "the salt of the earth." If you have a Kapha for a friend they will likely be there through thick and thin, showing up with a quiet presence when you most need them.

When *in balance* Kaphas are calm, steady, nurturing, stable, patient, and graceful. They often like working in the elements and with their hands. They make nurturing parents, loyal workers, dedicated researchers, artists, teachers, and farmers. When *out of balance*, Kaphas can get depressed, unmotivated, possessive, and lethargic.

A person with a predominant Kapha Dosha may experience health issues such as respiratory ailments, colds and excess mucus, sluggishness, stiffness, weak digestion, poor circulation, propensity to gain weight and retain water, and propensity for depression (especially in winter months). Kapha affects the lungs, heart, circulation, immunity, and energy levels.

BALANCING THE DOSHAS

Ayurveda recognizes that the first step in the disease process is our break from nature. Therefore, the very first intervention when there is an imbalance is to gently ask the dosha or the element that is disturbed to come back into balance. In other words, pray to the dosha. This helps us become aware of the natural elements of that dosha, so we can begin to find our way back into harmony with nature. For example, if you notice the fire element seems a bit out of balance because you have been losing your temper over small things, you could pause and sit for a moment and acknowledge the power and importance of the fire element in your life. Thankful for its light and heat, let that gratitude fill your heart. Humbly ask for this element to return to balance in your own body and life so you can fulfill your duties and be in relation with others in a loving and peaceful way. This brings conscious awareness to your relationship with the element.

When trying to balance each of the doshas, it is best to cultivate the opposite qualities of the doshas. For example, to balance Vata (the air element), it's helpful to focus on becoming grounded and steady, balancing mobility with stability. Pitta (the fire element) can achieve balance with practices that are cooling and calming, balancing hot and fiery with cool and calm. Kapha (the earth and water element) can turn to stimulation and movement for balance, balancing heaviness with lightness.

There are many small lifestyle changes that you can make to help bring your dosha back into balance, such as food choices, daily activities, exercise, and sleep habits. Additionally, to further help support harmony and balance, the introduction of herbs and detoxification practices can be used, although these are generally best prescribed by an Ayurvedic physician. Below you will find dosha-specific lifestyle choices, in which small changes can create large shifts.

Vata-Balancing Lifestyle Choices

If you are a primary Vata Dosha, you may want to consider the following suggestions to balance the wind and ether elements within you:

- Keep yourself warm.
- Consume warm food with some oil or ghee.
- Avoid raw food, cold drinks, and ice cream.
- Take small breaks during work.
- Keep a regular schedule and routine.
- Sleep properly (go to bed by 10 p.m.).
- Self-massage with warm sesame oil.
- Practice gentle yoga movements, breathing, relaxation, and meditation.
- Live with others whenever possible.

Foods: Vatas do best when eating regularly scheduled meals with some snacks between, and their foods need to be warm and moist, rather than dry or cold. Root vegetables are quite grounding for Vata. Veggies such as squash, beets, yams, and carrots are balancing for them. They may also enjoy avocados, peas, and asparagus, to name just a few. They do well with most grains such as rice, barley, oats, and quinoa. They can eat some of the small beans such as red lentils, split moong, whole moong, and even tofu, but beans can cause gas in Vata types since they are windy already, so it's best to combine beans and grains to reduce the probability of gas. They need some oils such as ghee or sunflower oil since they are dry by nature. They can eat fresh cheeses and eggs if they are not vegan. They do best with spices that are warming and stimulate digestion like salt and turmeric, cumin and coriander, fenugreek, and ginger. They can eat stewed fruits and do well with most fruits. They don't fare well with chips and crackers since they are too dry.

Activities: Vata types love to be busy and creative. They just need to try to stay focused, so they don't get too distracted. They can easily spin out, so finding ways to put a start time and a stop time to their activities helps them gather their energy.

Exercise: Vata types need to do strength building and grounding exercises. Additionally, working with yoga practices will help pacify the nervous system since Vata types are prone to anxiety.

Sleep: Vatas do best going to bed by 10 p.m. and getting up by 6 or 7 a.m. They sleep best when covered with a weighted blanket or being tucked in, providing them with a sense of grounding and security for the nervous system.[2]

Pitta-Balancing Lifestyle Choices

If you are a primary Pitta Dosha, you may want to consider the following suggestions to balance the fire and water elements within you:

- Moderation in life.
- Eat foods that are cooling (but cooked).
- Eat on time and take a snack in the afternoon.
- Don't overdo it. Rest.
- Exercise during the cool part of the day.
- Relax the eyes and don't overdo computers or screens.
- Develop compassion.
- Keep yourself cool and avoid direct sunlight.

- Practice gentle movements, breathing, relaxation, and meditation.

Foods: Pittas do best when they eat regular meals. They can get "hangry" quite easily if they miss meals. Leafy greens like kale, dandelion greens, beet greens, lettuce, and spinach help keep Pitta cool and breezy. They also do well with vegetables like broccoli, cauliflower, green beans, beets, and zucchini, and sweeter grains like basmati rice, quinoa, wheat, spelt, and barley are best. Pittas can eat some of the bigger beans since they have a stronger digestive fire than the other doshas, including navy beans, garbanzos, black beans, kidney beans, and lentils. The oils that suit them are coconut oil, olive oil, and ghee. If they are not vegan, they do well with egg whites, yogurt, and buttermilk. Fresh yogurt also helps cool Pitta. Being vegetarian or vegan can also help them develop compassion and kindness for all beings, which is especially good for Pitta since they can tend toward aggression when they are out of balance. The cooling spices like fennel, dill, coriander, saffron, cumin, and turmeric help cool their fiery nature and digestion. Sweet fruits like berries, peaches, grapes, and cherries help pacify their need for a sweet taste.

Activities: Pittas do best to not push it with their activities. Taking slow walks in nature, practicing simple yoga stretches, not competing in their work life or home life, and really making room for others to shine allows them to shine. While they are natural leaders, they need to also learn to be community minded. This might mean helping others by volunteering or reaching out to others in need.

Exercise: Pitta people need to be careful not to overexercise or overexert themselves since they naturally run hot. They are athletic and can get highly competitive with themselves and others. This can be tempered by choosing to participate in things like swimming or dancing or yoga, so they can enjoy movement without becoming too hot or too pushy with themselves or others. A nice moonlit walk or a walk in the cool part of the day is best for Pitta.

Sleep: Pitta needs to eat enough at dinnertime so they don't go to bed hungry. They do best going to bed before 10 p.m. and waking up by 6 or 7 a.m. Doing a gentle relaxation exercise before they fall off to sleep will help them calm down and sleep deeper. They do best to stay away from screens for several hours before bed since the light aggravates their fire element and keeps the mind engaged and hot.

Kapha-Balancing Lifestyle Choices

If you are a primary Kapha Dosha, you may want to consider the following suggestions to balance the earth and water elements within you:

- Wake up early and don't nap during the day.
- Stimulate the senses.
- Try new things to break routines and challenge yourself.
- Clear your space to avoid clutter.
- Reduce water consumption.
- Exercise vigorously (Kaphas do well to sweat).
- Use of light or heat therapy.
- Avoid cold drinks, ice cream, and sweets.
- Consume light food with lots of fresh vegetables, herbs, and spices.
- Eat less and fast one day a week.
- Stay warm and avoid dampness.

Foods: Cooked leafy greens like mustard greens, spinach, and kale are light and nourishing for Kapha types. Okra, sprouts, broccoli, cauliflower, and peppers will also help balance Kapha.

Some grains include buckwheat, amaranth, quinoa, corn, and millet. They do well with beans like aduki beans, black beans, mung beans, white beans, tofu, and tempeh. Oils should be taken in small amounts. Ghee, sunflower oil, and flaxseed oil are just a few that can be used. Kapha types do well as vegetarians or vegans. Fruits like pomegranates, strawberries, apples, cranberries, persimmons, and raspberries are good choices for Kapha. Lastly, they do well with hot spices that help dry up some of the excess water they have, such as chilis, mustard seeds, garlic, ginger, cumin, black pepper, cinnamon, and cloves. Kapha types need to eat less than the other types since they are prone to slow digestion that leaves them carrying extra weight. They should be careful not to drink ice water since it dampens and lowers their digestive fire. They even need to be aware of not drinking too much water, since their constitution is quite damp to begin with and they can tend to hold onto water.

Activities: Kapha types need to stay busy and keep trying new things to stimulate their senses—even something as simple as taking a new route to and from work each day. They need to avoid falling into a rut or becoming too routinized. Sometimes they need a Vata type to run them around and keep pushing them to try new things. Having pets can ensure they get outside to exercise since their love for animals will outweigh their desire to stay in bed or curled up with a good book.

Exercise: Kapha types need a lot of exercise to keep their fire burning. They need to work hard and generate a sweat to help move the sluggish and heavy nature of the water and earth elements. Running, walking fast, dancing, swimming, Zumba, flow yoga, hot yoga, and pickleball are great examples. Practicing any sports that they enjoy will be helpful in getting them to move more.

Sleep: Kapha needs to sleep less than the other doshas, because of their propensity to get depressed and heavy. Sleeping too long or day sleeping makes them feel much worse. Staying up until 10 or 11 p.m. and getting up early before the sun comes up, at 5 or 6 a.m., seems to give them the most sustainable energy.

As you read through the different body types and their qualities, you may have noticed that you resonated with some of them more than others. We all have varying degrees of all these elements, so there are many practices like those in this book that help bring balance to all the doshas. Those practices that balance all the doshas are called *tridoshic practices.* Practices like gentle movements, relaxation, meditation, breathing, and imagery help balance the three doshas. Keep in mind that during the seasons that these doshas belong to, we will be more affected by them. This is to say, in summer, Pitta (the fire and water dosha) is more predominant outside, and therefore it will be more active in our own bodies. Vata (the air and space dosha) is more predominant in the fall, when the winds are strong. Kapha (the earth and water element) is more predominant in the winter and spring. We can align with the doshas in this way, by making sure to honor the practices and activities that help balance the doshas in their corresponding seasons.

In addition to the dosha-balancing suggestions earlier, there are several practices that help keep the body and mind in tune with nature. These practices can be used by anyone, at any time, to bring them back into harmony with the natural world. As you introduce these practices into your life, trust that whatever connection to nature you are called to is the right one for you. Here are just a few practices to consider.

HARMONIZING WITH THE ELEMENTS
Earth Element Practices
Forest Bathing

Not only does walking in nature feel good, but there is real evidence to show that it relieves stress and supports mental health.[3] The practice of *shinrin-yoku*, also known as forest bathing, which gained popularity in the 1950s in Japan, is an effective way to reduce stress. It involves mindful walking in the forest while taking in the energy and healing benefits of nature. Many people love to hike, but forest bathing asks us to be more intentional with our steps. It teaches us to look around and soak in the beauty and energy all around us.

Hiking

Hiking can also be an inspiring way to take in nature and connect to the earth, if you can let go of the goal of trying to get somewhere or see something at the end of your hike. Try mindful hiking with a broader awareness and willingness to drop into the moment while taking in the beauty that surrounds you.

Walking Barefoot on the Earth

In addition to forest bathing and hiking is the practice of walking barefoot on the earth. There are many electrons available to us through the connection of our feet to the earth. Our ancestors lived with their feet on the earth every day, but since the invention of rubber-soled shoes we have less access to the healing properties of these electrons than we did with breathable leather soles. When we walk barefoot, we take in those electrons along with the energy (prana) from the earth through our feet. This is also known as *earthing*. Research shows that *earthing* can lower inflammation markers and reduce stress while having positive effects on the immune system, sleep, and even heart rate variability.[4] It doesn't require much time or even a forest to walk in. You can do it for a few minutes in a park or in your own yard if you have one. Even a short practice of walking meditation outside (outlined in chapter 5) can bring you back into harmony with the healing properties of the earth.

Gardening

Gardening not only puts your hands back in the dirt and your body back in the elements, but it puts you in direct connection to the plants that nourish us. All plants take in the carbon dioxide we breathe out, and we breathe in the oxygen the plants breathe out. Our lives are interdependent. Additionally, connecting to the process of growing plants for food is central to health and healing. What goes into the food goes into us. This includes the soil the plants grow in, the water from the rain, the light and heat from the sun, and the wind that blows and strengthens the plants while spreading seeds around to assist in germination.

Water Element Practices
Swimming

Swimming is an invigorating way to connect with the water element. If you are fortunate enough to have a lake, a pond, or even an ocean nearby, these natural bodies of water make an excellent source of connection to the water element. Even walking on the shore or dipping your feet in as you walk imparts a sense of communion with the water element.

Waterfalls

Waterfalls are a breathtaking wonder in the natural world and a source of enormous amounts of negative ions, which are produced by the sheer energy of falling and moving water. Research on these negative ions has shown that they have a positive and powerful effect on minimizing the symptoms of depression.[5] There is a similar effect when standing on the shore as waves crash in.

Hot Springs

People have sought out soaking in natural hot springs for centuries. Hot springs are known for their effects on the skin and for lowering stress levels, and they continue to be a place for those looking for rejuvenation. When I was traveling in England, we spent a day exploring the city of Bath, known for its Roman baths and sulfur hot springs, built in AD 75. I was impressed by the way the whole town used to organize around these healing waters for their stress-relieving qualities. To this day, the site is a must-see for tourists traveling through the area to feel the powerful energy these springs once held, and to remember how our ancestors used to converse with the water element.

Fire Element Practices
Sitting Around a Fire

Allowing the hypnotic pull of the flames to draw you into a fire's warm embrace is one way to create a relationship with the fire element. There is something so transfixing about a fire. While gazing at the intense light from the flames, it's hard to turn away. Fire is transformative. It transforms light into images so we can see. In the stomach, the fire element transforms food into energy, and in the mind, it enlightens our thought process.

Sunrises and Sunsets

Watching a sunrise or sunset is yet another irresistible expression of the fire element. Without the sun we would not exist. There is an awe that hangs in the air as the sun rises and sets. It is a significant marker to the beginning and end of each day on this planet and allows us to fully feel our connection to the fire element.

Air Element Practices
Bird-Watching

Not only is bird-watching captivating and relaxing, but it also gifts us the opportunity to unite with the air element. The grace and beauty of birds in flight awakens us to our own ethereal and airy nature. In some traditions, the birds are said to connect us to the heavens. Many cultures believe that our departed loved ones visit us as birds. They are like messengers from the other side. Have you ever noticed a synchronistic encounter with a bird right after losing a loved one? I can recall several visits of my own. My mother-in-law came to me as an owl the night she passed, and my aunt and uncle as playful cardinals on the day of my aunt's burial. My own father has come as a yellow finch and a cardinal to remind me he is close during difficult times. There are no words spoken, just a felt sense, a deep knowingness, and a feeling of support and spiritual significance when they show up.

Kite Flying

Kite flying is another way to connect to the air element. For a kite to fly, it requires a sensitivity to just the right amount of lift and pull on the kite string to send it soaring. Our own energy seems to be lifted up as we raise our gaze to follow the graceful flow of the kite. We can actually feel the pull and the force of the currents in our fingers as we navigate its flight. Once the kite takes flight, there is something quite uplifting and exhilarating about connecting to the air element in this way.

Ether (Space) Element Practices
Cloud Watching

As children, many of us remember lying on our backs somewhere in nature watching the cloud formations. Almost like a Rorschach test, we all saw something different in their shapes. More importantly, we were transported to the world of space. As we rest our gaze on the clouds and then the space between them, the mind becomes more spacious and open. We lose our sense of boundaries and can see things from a much broader perspective. This kind of expansiveness is necessary for our spirit to feel nourished and held.

Star Gazing

From the beginning of time people have looked to the stars for wisdom and guidance, and to the vast universe for answers and inspiration. We have a deep connection to the stars and the solar system; as planetary scientist and stardust expert Dr. Ashley King explains, "Most of the elements of our bodies were formed in stars over the course of billions of years and multiple star lifetimes.

However, it's also possible that some of our hydrogen (which makes up roughly 9.5 percent of our bodies) and lithium, which our body contains in very tiny trace amounts, originated from the Big Bang."[6] We have quite literally descended from the stars, so of course we feel that connection.

The science of astronomy and astrology are both ways we have tried to find scientific meaning from the stars, planets, and worlds around us. In today's world we look down at our phones, fixing our gaze and narrowing our focus to tune into the information and connection our phones provide. As a result, our view and vision has narrowed. When we look to the stars, we align with the infinite. We see ourselves as both vast and specific. Looking into space our individual consciousness begins to spread out, giving us the experience of being part of something much bigger than ourselves.

Finding a way to connect with all the elements is what heals us. It brings us back to our roots and puts us right in the middle of nature.

Cooking and Eating as a Way to Join with Nature

Another important way we can connect to all the elements of nature is through mindful cooking and eating practices. Everything we consume is absorbed and assimilated into what becomes the building blocks of the physical body, as well as the vibrational frequency of the energetic body. Therefore, what and how we eat becomes vital to our health and healing.

It is important, whenever possible, to eat foods that are fresh, organic, local, and of the highest quality, carrying the highest vibrational energy or prana. Fresh foods that have been well attended to while they are grown have a different vibration than foods that are not farmed with that same attention. In addition, foods that are boxed, frozen, or canned don't carry the same vibrational energy as freshly cooked foods. Keep in mind that foods that are nutrient-dense and align with the suggestions for your specific dosha will be the most nourishing.

It is a privilege to have access to the highest-quality foods, and sometimes this is not possible. In that case remember that your mindset can play an important role in receiving the most value from your foods. Setting an intention that the foods you are eating are blessed and nourishing will have a positive effect on your digestion and assimilation.

Foods have prana, life force. When we cook, we are touching the food and imbuing it with our energy. What we put into the food, we get back from the food. When I lived in the yoga institute, I worked in and managed the vegetarian kitchen. We practiced meditation in action as we prepared the food, and there was an intention of putting love and energy into the foods as we cooked for the community. We understood that if we cooked with a calm and peaceful presence, the food would have a calming effect on those who would eat it. We would put mindful attention to chopping, grinding, and stirring by hand, and would avoid using loud food grinders and choppers whenever possible to create a more peaceful environment around the food.

I remember several times while working in the kitchen, the swami would refuse the food if there had been any kind of disharmony in the kitchen that day. This kind of sensitivity to food helps us recognize that it's not just what we eat but even the circumstances around us while we cook and eat that contribute to the vitality of our foods. Eating on the run or when we are stressed or angry will most certainly affect our digestion. We all can feel the difference when we eat a meal that was prepared with the freshest ingredients. We can all taste the difference when a meal is made with heart-centered attention and love. One of my favorite spots to eat is a Vietnamese vegan restaurant run by Buddhist nuns. You can hear them singing prayers over the food as they cook, and every bite feels like a blessing.

Taking time to pray or send gratitude to all the people involved in growing, harvesting, delivering, and cooking our foods will keep us in contact with the cycle of food from seedling to stomach (see the mindful eating exercise in chapter 5). This kind of recognition of all that has gone into your food is one of the greatest digestive enzymes you have.

Finding Our Way Back

Since we have moved to an agrarian way of life and away from the hunter/gatherer societies of the past, we have stepped further and further away from our connection to nature. In today's world it is easy to lose our connection to food because we have lost our connection to nature. If you ask children where the chicken tenders or hamburger they just ate came from, many will look bewildered and say, "the refrigerator." They don't know what animals or vegetables they are even eating. That's why I am so encouraged to hear about the many programs, especially some of the inner-city school programs, that introduce children to gardening and cooking at the elementary level. This kind of introduction will stay with them for a lifetime and will provide more education about healthy food choices and living a healthy life in connection to nature and the elements. As we bring back the local farmers markets and backyard gardens, we are finding our way back into a relationship to our roots, so to speak.

We are beings that are born out of nature and its elements. We are a part of something much bigger than just our individual being and individual consciousness. We are quite literally part of nature. Remembering our connection to the natural world allows us the privilege of seeing ourselves as part of something bigger, gifting us a wider, more spacious view that helps us understand the importance of our place in the diverse landscape of this universe.

"You are comprised of 84 minerals, 23 elements, and 8 gallons of water spread across 38 trillion cells. You have been built up from nothing by the spare parts of the Earth you have consumed, according to a set of instructions hidden in a double helix and small enough to be carried by a sperm. You are recycled butterflies, plants, rocks, streams, firewood, wolf fur, and shark teeth, broken down to their smallest parts and rebuilt into our planet's most complex living thing. You are not living on Earth. You are Earth."

—AUBREY MARCUS[7]

Chapter 9

Unity

Bringing It All Together

"If you don't work out, sleep, meditate, relax, or do whatever special things you need to do for you, you won't be the best version of yourself. When you're not your best version of yourself, you can't do things for others. In a way, it's actually selfless to take great care of yourself because it allows you to be more present for your family and friends."

—HEATHER MONAHAN[1]

A CENTERING MOMENT

Affirming Your Daily Self-Care Practices

- Sit quietly in a comfortable position.
- Take a deep, slow inhale breath and a long, slow exhale breath.
- Allow yourself to be still for a moment as you breathe normally.

- Now imagine a feeling of excitement, knowing you have a time set aside just for you to practice self-care today.
- Begin to imagine yourself starting your day with your daily stress management routine.
- Imagine the spot in your home that you have created for your practice. Notice the way you have set it up and how inviting and comfortable it feels.
- Know that this time is just for you, and you can choose whatever routine feels right for your body and mind today.
- Ask yourself, "What practices does my body need or want today?" Then listen to your inner wisdom and your own intuition.
- In your mind's eye, see yourself gracefully moving through the practices.
- Imagine being fully present to yourself throughout the practice.
- As you see the practice coming to an end, notice how your body feels.
- Know that you can return to this practice each day as a place of refuge and inspiration, and the effects will be cumulative.
- Sit quietly knowing that you are doing something good for yourself.
- Allow this imagery practice to serve as encouragement and motivation for your daily practice.

TRYING TO PRACTICE STRESS MANAGEMENT TECHNIQUES IN THE middle of a stressful situation is a bit like taking swimming lessons when you are drowning. These practices are meant to be practiced regularly each day as training. We practice each day so that when stressful situations arise, we respond differently. The more you practice, the more refined and nuanced the practice becomes. At some point your nervous system responds differently to stressful situations. One of the things I hear over and over again from people who do these practices daily is "Things that used to bother me, just don't bother me anymore" or "I don't seem to find myself in as many stressful situations." This is because the practices are informing your nervous system in new ways. You are building a foundation of strength and resilience.

You may be asking yourself, where do I go from here? How do I decide what to do? This book is like a menu of stress management options. When the techniques are woven together into a balanced practice, they create a profound pathway to health and healing. To help you get started, I have outlined different levels of practice and routines to go with them. I have also put together some practice sessions according to time frames, including some routines for better sleep.

In the beginning, it may be helpful to choose from the set routines created in this chapter for your convenience. Once you are familiar with some of the practices, you can begin to mix and match and create your own unique daily practice. Everyone is different, and your situation and level of need may vary based on your individual health and any challenges you face.

When putting a stress management practice together for yourself, it's important to first consider:

- Am I trying to slow, stop, or reverse a disease process?
- Would I like to use these practices as prevention?
- How much time do I want to dedicate to my practices each day?

With these questions in mind, it may be helpful for you to identify the level of practice that will best support you and your health goals.

LEVEL I (60–90 MINUTES PER DAY, 7 DAYS PER WEEK)

This level of practice is good for those who are:

- Wanting to stop or reverse heart disease or other lifestyle illnesses. Research shows that these practices should be done in combination with other lifestyle changes including a low-fat plant-based diet, moderate daily exercise, and love and support as outlined in *Undo It!* by Dr. Dean and Anne Ornish.[2]
- Dealing with high levels of stress in their life.
- Needing extra self-care due to physical illness or emotional challenges.
- Wanting to attain optimal health and healing outcomes.

When I worked with participants in Ornish Lifestyle Medicine, we observed that those who did more stress management practices (1.5–2 hours daily) in addition to the other lifestyle recommendations showed more reversal than those who did a minimum of 1 hour per day. While it may seem like a big investment of time, it is an investment in your well-being that pays off with feeling better.

LEVEL II (20–40 MINUTES PER DAY, 4–7 DAYS PER WEEK)

This level of practice is good for those who are:

- Wanting disease prevention practices.
- Wanting to maintain a regular practice but their time commitment may vary.

- Needing a moderate level of stress management support.
- Having trouble sleeping from stress-related issues.

LEVEL III (10–30 MINUTES, 1–7 DAYS PER WEEK)

This level of practice is best for those who are:

- Living with minimal stress in their lives but want a daily practice that supports a calm and peaceful life.
- Prefer doing short segments of practice throughout the day.
- Who want to add small practices throughout the day in addition to their Level I daily routine.
- Who don't have a regular practice but would like to have some stress management practices to introduce into their life.
- Needing a less structured way to practice stress management.

LEVEL IV (YOU CHOOSE THE AMOUNT OF TIME AND HOW MANY DAYS PER WEEK)

This level of practice is for those who:

- Like a more open practice that allows them to use their intuition as a guide.
- Want to mix and match practices as they go.
- Are not able to make a regular time commitment.

Once you have determined the level of practice that you would like to incorporate in your life, it's time to choose your routines. Below is a list of the practices discussed in earlier chapters that will be used to build the daily Centered Heart routines.

Gentle Movements (Chapter 2)
Warmups: Neck, Shoulders, Hands and Wrists, Feet and Ankles

Gentle Movements: Cobra, Half Locust, Crocodile, Seated Forward Bend, Seated Spinal Twist, Modified Shoulder Stand, Fish

Relaxation (Chapter 3)
Centering Relaxation, Deep Relaxation, Tense and Relax, Healing Imagery Practice Using Healing Light or Healing Energy

Breathing (Chapter 4)
Even Breathing, 2-to-1 Breathing, Abdominal Breathing, Long Wide and Deep Breathing, Three-Part Breathing, Alternate Nostril Breathing, Humming Breath

Meditation (Chapter 5)
Candle Gazing, Walking Meditation, Mindful Eating Practice, Breath-Centered Meditation, Meditation on a Word, Prayer, or Mantra, Meditation on a Feeling

Imagery (Chapter 6)
Specific Imagery Practice I, Specific Imagery Practice II, Non-Specific Imagery Practice, Imagining a Positive Outcome, Intention-Setting Practice

Cultivating Compassion (Chapter 7)
Meditation to Inspire Compassion, The Practice of Cultivating Compassion

Connecting to Nature (Chapter 8)
Harmonizing with the Earth Element, Harmonizing with the Water Element, Harmonizing with the Fire Element, Harmonizing with the Air Element, Harmonizing with the Ether Element, Cooking and Eating as a Way to Connect with Nature

CENTERED HEART ROUTINES
Seven-Day Practice Routine for Level I (60–90 minutes per day, 7 days per week)
Bold denotes a new practice.

Day 1

- **Centering relaxation** *(chapter 3)*
- **Warmups: neck, shoulders, hands and wrists, feet and ankles** *(chapter 2)*
- **Gentle movements: crocodile, cobra, half locust, seated forward bend, seated spinal twist, modified shoulder stand, fish** *(chapter 2)*
- **Tense and relax** *(chapter 3)*
- **Abdominal breathing, even breathing** *(chapter 4)*
- **Breath-centered meditation** *(chapter 5)*

Day 2

- Centering relaxation *(chapter 3)*
- Warmups: choose one *(chapter 2)*
- Gentle movements: crocodile, cobra, half locust, seated forward bend, seated spinal twist, modified shoulder stand, fish *(chapter 2)*
- **The practice of deep relaxation** *(chapter 3)*
- **Healing imagery practice using healing light or healing energy** *(chapter 3)*
- **Three-part breathing** *(chapter 4)*
- **Candle-gazing meditation** *(chapter 5)*

Day 3

- Centering relaxation *(chapter 3)*
- Gentle movements: crocodile, cobra, half locust, seated forward bend, seated spinal twist, modified shoulder stand, fish *(chapter 2)*
- The practice of deep relaxation *(chapter 3)*
- Healing imagery practice using healing light or healing energy *(chapter 3)*
- **2-to-1 breathing** *(chapter 4)*
- **Meditation on a word, prayer, or mantra** *(chapter 5)*
- **Intention-setting practice** *(chapter 6)*

Day 4

- Centering relaxation *(chapter 3)*
- Gentle movements: crocodile, cobra, half locust, seated forward bend, seated spinal twist, modified shoulder stand, fish *(chapter 2)*
- The practice of deep relaxation *(chapter 3)*
- Healing imagery practice using healing light or healing energy *(chapter 3)*
- **Three-part breathing** *(chapter 4)*
- **Candle-gazing meditation** *(chapter 5)*

Day 5

- Centering relaxation *(chapter 3)*

- Warmups: neck, shoulders, hands and wrists, feet and ankles *(chapter 2)*
- The practice of deep relaxation *(chapter 3)*
- **Specific imagery practice I** *(chapter 6)*
- **Alternate nostril breathing** *(chapter 4)*
- **Meditation to inspire compassion** *(chapter 7)*

Day 6

- Centering relaxation *(chapter 3)*
- Gentle movements: crocodile, cobra, half locust, seated forward bend, seated spinal twist, modified shoulder stand, fish *(chapter 2)*
- Tense and relax *(chapter 3)*
- **Non-specific imagery practice I** *(chapter 6)*
- **Humming breath** *(chapter 4)*
- **Meditation on a feeling** *(chapter 5)*

Day 7

- **Walking meditation** *(chapter 5)*
- Warmups: choose one *(chapter 2)*
- Gentle movements: cobra, half locust, crocodile, seated forward bend, seated spinal twist, modified shoulder stand, fish *(chapter 2)*
- The practice of deep relaxation *(chapter 3)*
- Choose one breathing practice *(chapter 4)*
- **The practice of cultivating compassion** *(chapter 7)*

Level I practice can also include:

- Mindful eating practice during the first 5 minutes of one of your meals each day *(chapter 5)*
- Incorporating a connection to nature through harmonizing with the elements *(chapter 8)*
- A 60-minute practice using the "Daily Routines by Time" in this chapter
- Any of the 10- or 20-minute practices throughout the day if you are interested in extending past the 60 minutes of recommended practice
- Practices for better sleep in the evening before bed

Seven-Day Practice Routine for Level II (20–40 minutes per day, 4–7 days per week)

The days can be arranged according to the time you want to spend each day.

Day 1 (30–40 minutes)

- Centering relaxation *(chapter 3)*
- Gentle movements: cobra, half locust, seated forward bend, seated spinal twist *(chapter 2)*
- The practice of deep relaxation *(chapter 3)*
- Healing imagery practice using healing light or healing energy *(chapter 3)*

Day 2 (25–30 minutes)

- Three-part breathing *(chapter 4)*

- Warmups: neck, shoulders, hands and wrists, feet and ankles *(chapter 2)*
- Alternate nostril breathing *(chapter 4)*
- Meditation on a word prayer or feeling *(chapter 5)*

Day 3 (40 minutes)

- Walking meditation *(chapter 5)*
- Gentle movements: cobra, half locust, seated forward bend, seated spinal twist, modified shoulder stand, fish *(chapter 2)*
- Tense and relax *(chapter 3)*
- Specific imagery practice I *(chapter 6)*

Day 4 (30–40 minutes)

- Gentle movements: modified shoulder stand, fish *(chapter 2)*
- Humming breath *(chapter 4)* while in fish
- Non-specific imagery practice *(chapter 6)* while in fish
- Meditation: choose the technique you like most *(chapter 5)*

Day 5 (40 minutes)

- Centering relaxation *(chapter 3)*
- Warmups: choose one *(chapter 2)*
- Gentle movements: cobra, half locust, seated forward bend, seated spinal twist *(chapter 2)*
- The practice of deep relaxation *(chapter 3)*

- The practice of cultivating compassion *(chapter 7)*

Day 6 (20 minutes)

- 2-to-1 breathing combined with alternate nostril breathing *(chapter 4)*
- Meditation on a word, prayer, or phrase

Day 7 (30 minutes)

- Gentle movements: modified shoulder stand, fish *(chapter 2)*
- Tense and relax *(chapter 3)*
- Alternate nostril breathing *(chapter 4)*

Level II practice can also include:

- A 20- to 40-minute practice using the "Daily Routines by Time" in this chapter
- Incorporating a connection to nature through harmonizing with the elements *(chapter 8)*

Suggested Practice Routines for Level III (10–30 minutes, 1–7 days per week)

When putting together a daily practice for Level III, you can choose different combinations from the "Daily Routines by Time." Try to create a well-rounded practice using a variety of techniques. You choose the time of day and amount of time that works best that day—it may be helpful to dedicate a specific time each day if you have trouble making it a priority. Be creative and enjoy the flow.

Suggested Practice Routines for Level IV (you choose the amount of time and how many days per week)

When putting together a daily practice for Level IV, it is important to honor what your body is telling you each day. Some people in Level IV will want to have a whole hour each day for practice and choose what practices to use based on how they are feeling that day. This is a very advanced and intuitive practice that can be cultivated with regular practice and awareness of your own specific body and needs.

DAILY ROUTINES BY TIME
10-Minute Practice Sessions

Set a timer for 10 minutes and choose one of the following practices for a quick reset:

- Alternate nostril breathing *(chapter 4)*
- Legs up on a chair in a modified shoulder stand and breathe as if your heart is breathing *(chapter 2)*
- Fish, add imagery of breathing from heart to feet and from hands to head *(chapter 2)*
- Walking meditation (barefoot on the earth optional) *(chapter 5)*
- Warmups: neck, shoulders, hands and wrists, feet and ankles *(chapter 2)*
- Meditation to inspire compassion *(chapter 7)*
- Imagining a positive outcome *(chapter 6)*
- Centering relaxation *(chapter 3)*
- Meditation on a candle flame *(chapter 5)*
- Humming breath, add 2-to-1 breathing to alternate nostril breathing *(chapter 4)*
- Intention-setting practice *(chapter 6)*

- Mindful eating practice *(chapter 5)*

20-Minute Practice Sessions

Set a timer for 20 minutes and choose one of the following practice sequences:

- Alternate nostril breathing *(chapter 4)*; meditation on a word prayer or mantra *(chapter 5)*
- Gentle movements: cobra, half locust, crocodile, seated forward bend, seated spinal twist, modified shoulder stand, fish *(chapter 2)*; humming breath while in fish pose *(chapter 4)*
- Tense and relax *(chapter 3)*; healing imagery practice *(chapter 3)*
- Warmups: neck, shoulders, hands and wrists, feet and ankles *(chapter 2)*; the practice of cultivating compassion *(chapter 7)*
- Centering relaxation *(chapter 3)*; gentle movements: modified shoulder stand, fish *(chapter 2)*; 2-to-1 breathing while in fish pose *(chapter 4)*
- Alternate nostril breathing *(chapter 4)*; warmups: neck, shoulders, hands and wrists, feet and ankles *(chapter 2)*; the practice of deep relaxation *(chapter 3)*
- Gentle movements: cobra, half locust, seated forward bend, seated spinal twist *(chapter 2)*, alternate nostril breathing *(chapter 4)*; meditation on a feeling *(chapter 5)*
- Fish pose with imagery practice breathing from heart to feet and from hands to head *(chapter 2)*; humming breath *(chapter 4)*

60-Minute Practice Sessions

Set a timer for 60 minutes and choose one of the following practice sessions:

Practice Session 1

- Centering relaxation *(chapter 3)*
- Abdominal breathing, even breathing *(chapter 4)*
- Warmups: neck, shoulders, hands and wrists, feet and ankles *(chapter 2)*
- Gentle movements: crocodile, cobra, half locust, seated forward bend, seated spinal twist, modified shoulder stand, fish *(chapter 2)*
- Tense and relax *(chapter 3)*
- Healing imagery practice using healing light or healing energy *(chapter 3)*
- Breath-centered meditation *(chapter 5)*

Practice Session 2

- Centering relaxation *(chapter 3)*
- Abdominal breathing, even breathing *(chapter 4)*
- Warmups: choose one *(chapter 2)*
- Gentle movements: crocodile, cobra, half locust, seated forward bend, seated spinal twist, modified shoulder stand, fish *(chapter 2)*
- The practice of deep relaxation *(chapter 3)*
- Specific imagery practice I *(chapter 6)*
- 2-to-1 breathing *(chapter 4)*
- Alternate nostril breathing *(chapter 4)*

Practice Session 3

- Walking meditation *(chapter 5)*
- Gentle movements: crocodile, cobra, half locust, seated forward bend, seated spinal twist, modified shoulder stand, fish *(chapter 2)*
- Tense and relax *(chapter 3)*
- Healing imagery practice using healing light or healing energy *(chapter 3)*
- Humming breath *(chapter 4)*
- Meditation on a word, prayer, or mantra *(chapter 5)*

Practice Session 4

- Centering relaxation *(chapter 3)*
- Warmups: neck, shoulders, hands and wrists, feet and ankles *(chapter 2)*
- Gentle movements: modified shoulder stand, fish *(chapter 2)*
- The practice of deep relaxation *(chapter 3)*
- The practice of cultivating compassion *(chapter 7)*
- Three-part breathing *(chapter 4)*
- Breath-centered meditation *(chapter 5)*

Practice Session 5

- Three-part breathing *(chapter 4)*
- Alternate nostril breathing *(chapter 4)*
- Warmups: neck, shoulders, hands and wrists, feet and ankles *(chapter 2)*

- Gentle movements: crocodile, cobra, half locust, seated forward bend, seated spinal twist, modified shoulder stand, fish *(chapter 2)*
- Tense and relax *(chapter 3)* with healing imagery practice using healing light or healing energy *(chapter 3)*
- Meditation on a feeling *(chapter 5)*

Practice Session 6

- Centering relaxation *(chapter 3)*
- Gentle movements: crocodile, cobra, half locust, seated forward bend, seated spinal twist, modified shoulder stand, fish *(chapter 2)*
- The practice of deep relaxation *(chapter 3)*
- Specific imagery practice I *(chapter 6)*
- Meditation on a word, prayer, or mantra *(chapter 5)*

PRACTICE SESSIONS FOR BETTER SLEEP

Choose one of these gentle practices before bed to help unwind from the day and drift into restorative, healing sleep.

- The practice of deep relaxation *(chapter 3)*
- 1–2 minutes of abdominal breathing, 1–2 minutes of 2-to-1 breathing, followed by 1–2 minutes of humming breath *(chapter 4)*
- Tense and relax *(chapter 3)*
- 10–15 minutes of three-part breathing *(chapter 4)* with healing imagery practice using healing light or healing energy *(chapter 3)*
- 10–15 minutes of meditation on a candle flame *(chapter 5)*

- Fish pose *(chapter 2)* combined with 2-to-1 breathing, followed by humming breath *(chapter 4)*

MAKING STRESS MANAGEMENT A PRIORITY

"You should sit in meditation for 20 minutes a day, unless you're too busy. Then you should sit for an hour."

—ZEN PROVERB

THE BIGGEST CONCERN PEOPLE TELL ME THEY HAVE ABOUT introducing a stress management practice into their lives is finding time. Life seems full of things to do, and yet sometimes it feels like those things are doing us.

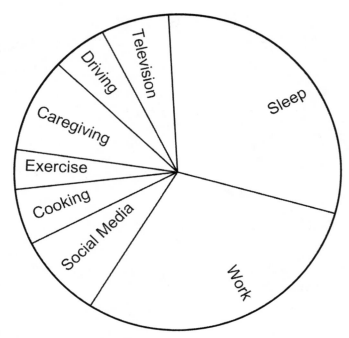

Figure 9.1. How Do I Spend My Time?

Though time is a man-made construct invented to help organize our lives, it also seems to be the biggest obstacle to our happiness and enjoyment. Some important questions to ask yourself: How am I currently using my time? Where is my energy going? What am I prioritizing in my life and does that priority serve me? It can be helpful to create a pie chart to help you visualize where you spend your time and energy.

Start by drawing a circle, then think about all the activities you do throughout the day that take up a significant amount of your time. Some examples include sleep, work, social media, television, gym/exercise, movement practices, reading, listening to podcasts or music, meditation, eating, time spent with friends and family, caring for others, caring for pets, school, studying, cooking, cleaning, shopping, sports, driving, and so on. Then separate your pie into individual slices that represent and correspond with how much time you spend doing each activity.

Once you have drawn your pie and can visualize your time, check in to see if everything in your pie is something you need or want in your life. Next, ask yourself if the time you're spending on each activity is the time you would like to be spending on that activity. Recognize that you are making choices every day about what you want in your life and how you want to spend your time. Where we put our energy becomes our priority, and we make time for what we prioritize.

The stress management practices outlined in this book help inform how you view and experience everything in your life. They allow you to make conscious choices about what and who you want to be in any given circumstance. They also set the foundation for your own self-care and healing. By putting your own health first, it allows you to bring your best self to your life and to the lives of others.

One way to make these practices a priority is rather than trying to squeeze them into your already busy life, allow your life to take shape around your daily practices. Dedicate yourself to your own self-care with a daily practice that has been proven to reduce stress by changing the way you react to stressful situations. As you practice, the evidence for these practices is informed by your own experience.

Life's circumstances can leave us feeling like we are forever on a wheel of ups and downs that is dictated by what happens outside of us. While sometimes it may not feel that way, the way we react to what happens is a choice. These practices lengthen the space between action and reaction to provide a powerful pause. That pause allows us the freedom to choose how we want to respond and who we want to be. Those small decisions shape our lives and who we are. They are key to our own peace and happiness. When we are calm and centered, everything looks different than when we are stressed and disorganized. Clarity and discernment then rise to the surface, and our path becomes clear.

Living with a centered heart isn't about getting rid of all the stressors in your life, as that's impossible. It's about finding ways to best support yourself to be able to deal and cope with those stressors. It's about finding your way back. Back to yourself, back to your health, back to your heart.

May there be peace in your body, peace in your mind, and peace in your heart.

May all beings know peace.

Om Shanti, Shanti, Shanti.

Peace, Peace, and only Peace.

NOTES

INTRODUCTION

1. Parker, Stephen. "Training Attention for Conscious Non-REM Sleep: The Yogic Practice of Yoga-Nidrā and Its Implications for Neuroscience Research." *Progress in Brain Research*, 2019, 255–72. https://doi.org/10.1016/bs.pbr.2018.10.016.

2. Ornish, D., S. E. Brown, J. H. Billings, L. W. Scherwitz, W. T. Armstrong, T. A. Ports, S. M. McLanahan, R. L. Kirkeeide, K. L. Gould, and R. J. Brand. "Can Lifestyle Changes Reverse Coronary Heart Disease?" *The Lancet* 336, no. 8708 (July 22, 1990): 129–33. https://doi.org/10.1016/0140-6736(90)91656-u.

3. Ornish, Dean. "Avoiding Revascularization with Lifestyle Changes: The Multicenter Lifestyle Demonstration Project." *American Journal of Cardiology* 82, no. 10 (November 26, 1998): 72–76. https://doi.org/10.1016/s0002-9149(98)00744-9.

CHAPTER 1

1. Frankl, Viktor. *Man's Search for Meaning*. Boston, MA: Beacon Press, 2006.

2. "Heart Disease Facts." Centers for Disease Control and Prevention, October 14, 2022. https://www.cdc.gov/heartdisease/facts.htm.

3. Dimsdale, Joel. "Psychological Stress and Cardiovascular Disease." *Journal of the American College of Cardiology* 51, no. 13 (April 1, 2008): 1237–46. https://doi.org/https://doi.org/10.1016/j.jacc.2007.12.024.

4. Chu, Paula, Rinske A. Gotink, Gloria Y. Yeh, Sue J. Goldie, and M. G. Myriam Hunink. "The Effectiveness of Yoga in Modifying Risk Factors for Cardiovascular Disease and Metabolic Syndrome: A Systematic Review and Meta-Analysis of Randomized Controlled Trials." *European Journal of Preventive Cardiology* 23, no. 3 (2014): 291–307. https://doi.org/10.1177/2047487314562741.

5. Srihari Sharma, K. N., NidhiRam Choudhary, and Pailoor Subramanya. "Evidence Base of Yoga Studies on Cardiovascular Health: A Bibliometric

Analysis." *International Journal of Yoga* 12, no. 2 (May 6, 2019): 162. https://doi
.org/10.4103/ijoy.ijoy_6_18.

6. Bhavanani, Ananda Balayogi. "Role of Yoga in Prevention and Management
of Lifestyle Disorders." *Yoga Mimamsa* 49, no. 2 (December 17, 2017): 42. https:
//doi.org/10.4103/ym.ym_14_17.

7. Bhavanani, Ananda Balayogi, and Meena Ramanathan. "Immediate Cardiovascular Effects of a Single Yoga Session in Different Conditions." *Alternative
& Integrative Medicine* 02, no. 09 (2013). https://doi.org/10.4172/2327-5162
.1000144.

CHAPTER 2

1. Hashmi, Hina. *Your Life: A Practical Guide to Happiness Peace and Fulfilment.*
Memphis, TN: For Betterment Publications, 2014.

2 Bhavanani, Ananda Balayogi, and Meena Ramanathan. "Immediate Cardiovascular Effects of a Single Yoga Session in Different Conditions." *Alternative
& Integrative Medicine* 02, no. 09 (2013). https://doi.org/10.4172/2327-5162
.1000144.

3. Djalilova, Dilorom M., Paula S. Schulz, Ann M. Berger, Adam J. Case,
Kevin A. Kupzyk, and Alyson C. Ross. "Impact of Yoga on Inflammatory
Biomarkers: A Systematic Review." *Biological Research for Nursing* 21, no. 2
(2018): 198–209. https://doi.org/10.1177/1099800418820162.

4. "Integral Yoga® Teachings." Integral Yoga. Accessed March 16, 2023. https:
//integralyoga.org/teachings/.

CHAPTER 3

1. Harris, Sydney J. "Strictly Personal: You're Too Busy? Time to Relax." *Chicago Daily News*, October 26, 1954.

2. "Sleep Plays an Important Role in Heart Health." Heart.org, January 13,
2023. https://www.heart.org/en/health-topics/sleep-disorders/sleep-and-heart
-health.

3. Özlü, Ibrahim, Zeynep Öztürk, Zeynep Karaman Özlü, Erdal Tekin, and
Ali Gür. "The Effects of Progressive Muscle Relaxation Exercises on the Anxiety
and Sleep Quality of Patients with Covid-19: A Randomized Controlled Study."
Perspectives in Psychiatric Care 57, no. 4 (March 2, 2021): 1791–97. https://doi
.org/10.1111/ppc.12750.

4. Moszeik, Esther N., Timo von Oertzen, and Karl-Heinz Renner. "Effectiveness of a Short Yoga Nidra Meditation on Stress, Sleep, and Well-Being
in a Large and Diverse Sample." *Current Psychology* 41, no. 8 (September 8,
2020): 5272–86. https://doi.org/10.1007/s12144-020-01042-2.

5. Hyman, Mark. "Are You Suffering From Adrenal Dysfunction?" Video blog.
Dr. Hyman (blog). Accessed February 21, 2023.

6. Sundar, S., S. K. Agrawal, V. P. Singh, S. K. Bhattacharya, K. N. Udupa, and S. K. Vaish. "Role of Yoga in Management of Essential Hypertension." *Acta Cardiologica* 39, no. 3 (January 1, 1984): 203–8.

7. Mariotti, Agnese. "The Effects of Chronic Stress on Health: New Insights into the Molecular Mechanisms of Brain–Body Communication." *Future Science OA* 1, no. 3 (November 2015). https://doi.org/10.4155/fso.15.21.

8. "What Causes an Adrenaline Rush? The Impact of Epinephrine and Certain Situations." WebMD, April 27, 2021. https://www.webmd.com/a-to-z -guides/what-to-know-adrenaline-rush.

9. Damodaran, A., A. Malathi, N. Patil, N. Shah, Suryavansihi, and S. Marathe. "Therapeutic Potential of Yoga Practices in Modifying Cardiovascular Risk Profile in Middle Aged Men and Women." *Journal of the Association of Physicians of India* 50, no. 5 (May 1, 2002): 633–40.

10. Devi, Nischala Joy. *The Healing Path of Yoga: Time-Honored Wisdom and Scientifically Proven Methods That Alleviate Stress, Open Your Heart, and Enrich Your Life.* New York: Three Rivers Press, 2000.

CHAPTER 4

1. B. K. S. *Light on Yoga: The Bible of Modern Yoga.* New York, NY: Schocken, 1979.

2. "How Your Lungs Work." Lung Foundation Australia, December 9, 2022. https://lungfoundation.com.au/lung-health/protecting-your-lungs/how -your-lungs-work/.

3. Rowden, Adam. "Normal Respiration Rate: For Adults and All Ages, and How to Measure." *Medical News Today.* MediLexicon International, January 4, 2023. https://www.medicalnewstoday.com/articles/324409.

4. Mitchell, R. A., and A. J. Berger. "Neural Regulation of Respiration." *American Review of Respiratory Disease* 111, no. 2 (February 1, 1975). https://doi.org /10.1164/arrd.1975.111.2.206.

5. Bhavanani, Ananda Balayogi, Madanmohan, Zeena Sanjay, and Ishwar V. Basavaraddi. "Immediate Cardiovascular Effects of Pranava Pranayama in Hypertensive Patients." *Indian Journal of Physiology and Pharmacology* 56, no. 3 (July 2012): 273–78.

6. Malhotra, V., R. Bharshankar, N. Ravi, and O. L. Bhagat. "Acute Effects on Heart Rate Variability during Slow Deep Breathing." *Mymensingh Medical Journal* 30, no. 1 (January 2021): 208–13.

7. Bhavanani, Ananda Balayogi, Zeena Sanjay, and Madanmohan. "Immediate Effect of Sukha Pranayama on Cardiovascular Variables in Patients of Hypertension." *International Journal of Yoga Therapy* 21, no. 1 (2011): 73–76.

8. Adhana, Ritu, Rani Gupta, Jyoti Dvivedii, and Sohaib Ahmad. "The Influence of the 2:1 Yogic Breathing Technique on Essential Hypertension." *Indian Journal of Physiology and Pharmacology* 57, no. 1 (January 2013): 38–44.

9. Hendricks, Gay. *Conscious Breathing: Breathwork for Health, Stress Release, and Personal Mastery.* New York, NY: Bantam Books, 1995.

10. Pal, GopalKrushna, Ankit Agarwal, Shanmugavel Karthik, Pravati Pal, and Nivedita Nanda. "Slow Yogic Breathing through Right and Left Nostril Influences Sympathovagal Balance, Heart Rate Variability, and Cardiovascular Risks in Young Adults." *North American Journal of Medical Sciences* 6, no. 3 (March 2014): 145–51. https://doi.org/10.4103/1947-2714.128477.

CHAPTER 5

1. Chödrön, Pema. *When Things Fall Apart: Heart Advice for Difficult Times.* London, UK: Thorsons Classics, 2017.

2. Fioranelli, Massimo, Anna G. Bottaccioli, Francesco Bottaccioli, Maria Bianchi, Miriam Rovesti, and Maria G. Roccia. "Stress and Inflammation in Coronary Artery Disease: A Review Psychoneuroendocrineimmunology-Based." *Frontiers in Immunology* 9 (September 6, 2018). https://doi.org/10.3389/fimmu.2018.02031.

3. Levine, Glenn N., Richard A. Lange, C. Noel Bairey-Merz, Richard J. Davidson, Kenneth Jamerson, Puja K. Mehta, Erin D. Michos, et al. "Meditation and Cardiovascular Risk Reduction: A Scientific Statement from the American Heart Association." *Journal of the American Heart Association* 6, no. 10 (September 28, 2017). https://doi.org/10.1161/jaha.117.004176.

4. Koike, Marcia Kiyomi, and Roberto Cardoso. "Meditation Can Produce Beneficial Effects to Prevent Cardiovascular Disease." *Hormone Molecular Biology and Clinical Investigation* 18, no. 3 (June 2014): 137–43. https://doi.org/10.1515/hmbci-2013-0056.

5. "Mindfulness Definition: What Is Mindfulness." Greater Good. Accessed February 22, 2023. https://greatergood.berkeley.edu/topic/mindfulness/definition.

CHAPTER 6

1. Vonnegut, Kurt. *Mother Night.* London, UK: Vintage Digital, 2020.

2. Stephens, Rebecca. "Imagery." *Clinical Nurse Specialist* 7, no. 4 (July 1993): 170–74. https://doi.org/10.1097/00002800-199307000-00004.

3. Krau, Stephen D. "The Multiple Uses of Guided Imagery." *Nursing Clinics of North America* 55, no. 4 (December 2020): 467–74. https://doi.org/10.1016/j.cnur.2020.06.013.

4. Mane, Rekha Vishnu, and Shital Waghmare. "A Study to Assess the Impact of Guided Imagery Therapy on Blood Pressure among Hypertensive Geriatric Group Residing in Selected Old Age Home of Pune City." *International Journal of Health Sciences & Research* 6, no. 7 (July 2016): 228–36.

5. Khait, I., U. Obolski, Y. Yovel, and L. Hadany. "Sound Perception in Plants." *Seminars in Cell & Developmental Biology* 92 (August 2019): 134–38. https://doi.org/10.1016/j.semcdb.2019.03.006.

6. Feinberg, Cara. "The Placebo Phenomenon." *Harvard Magazine*, March 3, 2014. https://www.harvardmagazine.com/2013/01/the-placebo-phenomenon.

7. Shmerling, Robert H. "The Placebo Effect: Amazing and Real." Harvard Health, June 22, 2020. https://www.health.harvard.edu/blog/the-placebo-effect-amazing-and-real-201511028544.

CHAPTER 7

1. Dossey, Larry. "Compassion: Why It Matters in Healing." Unity, March 9, 2020. https://upray.unity.org/resources/articles/compassion-why-it-matters-healing.

2. Batt-Rawden, Samantha A., Margaret S. Chisolm, Blair Anton, and Tabor E. Flickinger. "Teaching Empathy to Medical Students." *Academic Medicine* 88, no. 8 (August 2013): 1171–77. https://doi.org/10.1097/acm.0b013e318299f3e3.

3. "The Center for Compassion and Altruism Research: Current Research." The Center for Compassion and Altruism Research and Education. Accessed February 27, 2023. http://ccare.stanford.edu/research/current-research/#firsttab.

4. King, Martin Luther. *A Gift of Love: Sermons from Strength to Love and Other Preachings.* Boston, MA: Beacon Press, 2012.

5. Desmond, Małgorzata A., Jakub G. Sobiecki, Maciej Jaworski, Paweł Płudowski, Jolanta Antoniewicz, Meghan K. Shirley, Simon Eaton, et al. "Growth, Body Composition, and Cardiovascular and Nutritional Risk of 5- to 10-y-Old Children Consuming Vegetarian, Vegan, or Omnivore Diets." *American Journal of Clinical Nutrition* 113, no. 6 (June 1, 2021): 1565–77. https://doi.org/10.1093/ajcn/nqaa445.

6. Joy, Melanie. *Why We Love Dogs, Eat Pigs, and Wear Cows: An Introduction to Carnism: The Belief System That Enables Us to Eat Some Animals and Not Others.* Newburyport, MA: Red Wheel, 2020.

7. "Feeling the Heat: Factory Farming and Climate Change." ASPCA, August 22, 2022. https://www.aspca.org/news/feeling-heat-factory-farming-and-climate-change.

8. Dinu, Monica, Rosanna Abbate, Gian Franco Gensini, Alessandro Casini, and Francesco Sofi. "Vegetarian, Vegan Diets and Multiple Health Outcomes: A Systematic Review with Meta-Analysis of Observational Studies." *Critical Reviews in Food Science and Nutrition* 57, no. 17 (November 13, 2017): 3640–49. https://doi.org/10.1080/10408398.2016.1138447.

9. Ornish, Dean, R. J. Brand, C. Hogeboom, R. L. Kirkeeide, T. A. Ports, W. T. Armstrong, S. Sparler, et al. "Intensive Lifestyle Changes for Reversal of Coronary Heart Disease." *JAMA* 280, no. 23 (December 16, 1998): 2001–7. https://doi.org/10.1001/jama.280.23.2001.

10. Ornish, Dean, and Anne Ornish. *Undo It!: How Simple Lifestyle Changes Can Reverse Most Chronic Diseases.* New York, NY: Ballantine Books, 2022.

11. Levine, Glenn N., Karen Allen, Lynne T. Braun, Hayley E. Christian, Erika Friedmann, Kathryn A. Taubert, Sue Ann Thomas, Deborah L. Wells, and

Richard A. Lange. "Pet Ownership and Cardiovascular Risk." *Circulation* 127, no. 23 (May 9, 2013): 2353–63. https://doi.org/10.1161/cir.0b013e31829201e1.

12. "2021–2022 APPA National Pet Owners Survey." American Pet Products Association. Accessed February 27, 2023. https://www.americanpetproducts.org/pubs_survey.asp.

13. "The Power of Pets." National Institutes of Health, U.S. Department of Health and Human Services, July 26, 2022. https://newsinhealth.nih.gov/2018/02/power-pets.

14. Nemeth, Maria. *Mastering Life's Energies: Simple Steps to a Luminous Life.* Novato, CA: New World Library, 2007.

15. Amendola, Susi. "Yoga Offers These Four Keys to Your Happiness." Ornish Lifestyle Medicine. Accessed February 27, 2023. https://www.ornish.com/zine/yoga-offers-these-four-keys-to-your-happiness/.

CHAPTER 8

1. Razani, Nooshin. "Prescribing Nature for Health." *TEDx Talks.* Lecture presented at the TEDx Nashville, June 14, 2016.

2. "4 Ways Weighted Blankets Can Actually Help You." Pennmedicine.org, March 24, 2022. https://www.pennmedicine.org/updates/blogs/health-and-wellness/2022/march/weighted-blankets.

3. Morita, E., S. Fukuda, J. Nagano, N. Hamajima, H. Yamamoto, Y. Iwai, T. Nakashima, H. Ohira, and T. Shirakawa. "Psychological Effects of Forest Environments on Healthy Adults: Shinrin-Yoku (Forest-Air Bathing, Walking) as a Possible Method of Stress Reduction." *Public Health* 121, no. 1 (January 2007): 54–63. https://doi.org/10.1016/j.puhe.2006.05.024.

4. Chevalier, Gaétan, Stephen T. Sinatra, James L. Oschman, Karol Sokal, and Pawel Sokal. "Earthing: Health Implications of Reconnecting the Human Body to the Earth's Surface Electrons." *Journal of Environmental and Public Health* 2012 (January 2012): 1–8. https://doi.org/10.1155/2012/291541.

5. Perez, Vanessa, Dominik D. Alexander, and William H. Bailey. "Air Ions and Mood Outcomes: A Review and Meta-Analysis." *BMC Psychiatry* 13, no. 1 (January 15, 2013). https://doi.org/10.1186/1471-244x-13-29.

6. Lotzof, Kerry. "Are We Really Made of Stardust?" Natural History Museum. Accessed February 27, 2023. https://www.nhm.ac.uk/discover/are-we-really-made-of-stardust.html.

7. Marcus, Aubrey. "What." *Aubrey Marcus* (blog), May 9, 2018. https://www.aubreymarcus.com/blogs/poetry/what.

CHAPTER 9

1. Monahan, Heather. *Confidence Creator.* Miami, FL: Boss in Heels, 2018.

2. Ornish, Dean, and Anne Ornish. *Undo It!: How Simple Lifestyle Changes Can Reverse Most Chronic Diseases.* New York, NY: Ballantine Books, 2022.

BIBLIOGRAPHY

Adhana, Ritu, Rani Gupta, Jyoti Dvivedii, and Sohaib Ahmad. "The Influence of the 2:1 Yogic Breathing Technique on Essential Hypertension." *Indian Journal of Physiology and Pharmacology* 57, no. 1 (January 2013): 38–44.

Amendola, Susi. "Yoga Offers These Four Keys to Your Happiness." Ornish Lifestyle Medicine. Accessed February 27, 2023. https://www.ornish.com /zine/yoga-offers-these-four-keys-to-your-happiness/.

Batt-Rawden, Samantha A., Margaret S. Chisolm, Blair Anton, and Tabor E. Flickinger. "Teaching Empathy to Medical Students." *Academic Medicine* 88, no. 8 (August 2013): 1171–77. https://doi.org/10.1097/acm .0b013e318299f3e3.

Bhavanani, Ananda Balayogi. "Role of Yoga in Prevention and Management of Lifestyle Disorders." *Yoga Mimamsa* 49, no. 2 (December 17, 2017): 42. https://doi.org/10.4103/ym.ym_14_17.

Bhavanani, Ananda Balayogi, and Meena Ramanathan. "Immediate Cardiovascular Effects of a Single Yoga Session in Different Conditions." *Alternative & Integrative Medicine* 02, no. 09 (2013). https://doi.org/10.4172/2327 -5162.1000144.

Bhavanani, Ananda Balayogi, Madanmohan, Zeena Sanjay, and Ishwar V. Basavaraddi. "Immediate Cardiovascular Effects of Pranava Pranayama in Hypertensive Patients." *Indian Journal of Physiology and Pharmacology* 56, no. 3 (July 2012): 273–78.

Bhavanani, Ananda Balayogi, Zeena Sanjay, and Madanmohan. "Immediate Effect of Sukha Pranayama on Cardiovascular Variables in Patients of Hypertension." *International Journal of Yoga Therapy* 21, no. 1 (2011): 73– 76. https://doi.org/10.17761/ijyt.21.1.y007g51341634172.

Chevalier, Gaétan, Stephen T. Sinatra, James L. Oschman, Karol Sokal, and Pawel Sokal."Earthing: Health Implications of Reconnecting the Human Body to the Earth's Surface Electrons." *Journal of Environmental and Public Health* 2012 (January 2012): 1–8. https://doi.org/10.1155/2012 /291541.

Chödrön, Pema. *When Things Fall Apart: Heart Advice for Difficult Times.* London: Thorsons Classics, 2017.

Chu, Paula, Rinske A. Gotink, Gloria Y. Yeh, Sue J. Goldie, and M. G. Myriam Hunink. "The Effectiveness of Yoga in Modifying Risk Factors for Cardiovascular Disease and Metabolic Syndrome: A Systematic Review and Meta-Analysis of Randomized Controlled Trials." *European Journal of Preventive Cardiology* 23, no. 3 (2014): 291–307. https://doi.org/10.1177/2047487314562741.

Damodaran, A., A. Malathi, N. Patil, N. Shah, Suryavansihi, and S. Marathe. "Therapeutic Potential of Yoga Practices in Modifying Cardiovascular Risk Profile in Middle Aged Men and Women." *Journal of the Association of Physicians of India* 50, no. 5 (May 1, 2002): 633–40.

Desmond, Małgorzata A., Jakub G. Sobiecki, Maciej Jaworski, Paweł Płudowski, Jolanta Antoniewicz, Meghan K. Shirley, Simon Eaton, et al. "Growth, Body Composition, and Cardiovascular and Nutritional Risk of 5- to 10-y-Old Children Consuming Vegetarian, Vegan, or Omnivore Diets." *American Journal of Clinical Nutrition* 113, no. 6 (June 1, 2021): 1565–77. https://doi.org/10.1093/ajcn/nqaa445.

Devi, Nischala Joy. *The Healing Path of Yoga: Time-Honored Wisdom and Scientifically Proven Methods That Alleviate Stress, Open Your Heart, and Enrich Your Life*. New York: Three Rivers Press, 2000.

Dimsdale, Joel. "Psychological Stress and Cardiovascular Disease." *Journal of the American College of Cardiology* 51, no. 13 (April 1, 2008): 1237–46. https://doi.org/https://doi.org/10.1016/j.jacc.2007.12.024.

Dinu, Monica, Rosanna Abbate, Gian Franco Gensini, Alessandro Casini, and Francesco Sofi. "Vegetarian, Vegan Diets and Multiple Health Outcomes: A Systematic Review with Meta-Analysis of Observational Studies." *Critical Reviews in Food Science and Nutrition* 57, no. 17 (November 13, 2017): 3640–49. https://doi.org/10.1080/10408398.2016.1138447.

Djalilova, Dilorom M., Paula S. Schulz, Ann M. Berger, Adam J. Case, Kevin A. Kupzyk, and Alyson C. Ross. "Impact of Yoga on Inflammatory Biomarkers: A Systematic Review." *Biological Research for Nursing* 21, no. 2 (2018): 198–209. https://doi.org/10.1177/1099800418820162.

Dossey, Larry. "Compassion: Why It Matters in Healing." Unity, March 9, 2020. https://upray.unity.org/resources/articles/compassion-why-it-matters-healing.

"Feeling the Heat: Factory Farming and Climate Change." ASPCA, August 22, 2022. https://www.aspca.org/news/feeling-heat-factory-farming-and-climate-change.

Feinberg, Cara. "The Placebo Phenomenon." *Harvard Magazine*, March 3, 2014. https://www.harvardmagazine.com/2013/01/the-placebo-phenomenon.

Fioranelli, Massimo, Anna G. Bottaccioli, Francesco Bottaccioli, Maria Bianchi, Miriam Rovesti, and Maria G. Roccia. "Stress and Inflammation in Coronary Artery Disease: A Review Psychoneuroendocrineimmunology-Based."

Frontiers in Immunology 9 (September 6, 2018). https://doi.org/10.3389/fimmu.2018.02031.

"4 Ways Weighted Blankets Can Actually Help You." Pennmedicine.org, March 24, 2022. https://www.pennmedicine.org/updates/blogs/health-and-wellness/2022/march/weighted-blankets.

Frankl, Viktor. *Man's Search for Meaning*. Boston, MA: Beacon Press, 2006.

Guina, Jeffrey, and Brian Merrill. "Benzodiazepines I: Upping the Care on Downers: The Evidence of Risks, Benefits and Alternatives." *Journal of Clinical Medicine* 7, no. 2 (2018): 17. https://doi.org/10.3390/jcm7020017.

Harris, Sydney J. "Strictly Personal: You're Too Busy? Time To Relax." *Chicago Daily News*. October 26, 1954.

Hashmi, Hina. *Your Life: A Practical Guide to Happiness, Peace and Fulfillment*. Memphis, TN: For Betterment Publications, 2014.

"Heart Disease Facts." Centers for Disease Control and Prevention, October 14, 2022. https://www.cdc.gov/heartdisease/facts.htm.

Hendricks, Gay. *Conscious Breathing: Breathwork for Health, Stress Release, and Personal Mastery*. New York: Bantam Books, 1995.

"How Your Lungs Work." Lung Foundation Australia, December 9, 2022. https://lungfoundation.com.au/lung-health/protecting-your-lungs/how-your-lungs-work/.

Hyman, Mark. "Are You Suffering from Adrenal Dysfunction?" Video blog. *Dr. Hyman* (blog). Accessed February 21, 2023. https://drhyman.com/blog/2017/05/26/suffering-adrenal-dysfunction/.

"Integral Yoga® Teachings." Integral Yoga. Accessed March 16, 2023. https://integralyoga.org/teachings/.

Iyengar, B. K. S. *Light on Yoga: The Bible of Modern Yoga*. New York: Schocken, 1979.

Joy, Melanie. *Why We Love Dogs, Eat Pigs, and Wear Cows: An Introduction to Carnism: The Belief System That Enables Us to Eat Some Animals and Not Others*. Newburyport, MA: Red Wheel, 2020.

Khait, I., U. Obolski, Y. Yovel, and L. Hadany. "Sound Perception in Plants." *Seminars in Cell & Developmental Biology* 92 (August 2019): 134–38. https://doi.org/10.1016/j.semcdb.2019.03.006.

King, Martin Luther. *A Gift of Love: Sermons from Strength to Love and Other Preachings*. Boston, MA: Beacon Press, 2012.

Koike, Marcia Kiyomi, and Roberto Cardoso. "Meditation Can Produce Beneficial Effects to Prevent Cardiovascular Disease." *Hormone Molecular Biology and Clinical Investigation* 18, no. 3 (June 2014): 137–43. https://doi.org/10.1515/hmbci-2013-0056.

Krau, Stephen D. "The Multiple Uses of Guided Imagery." *Nursing Clinics of North America* 55, no. 4 (December 2020): 467–74. https://doi.org/10.1016/j.cnur.2020.06.013.

Levine, Glenn N., Richard A. Lange, C. Noel Bairey-Merz, Richard J. Davidson, Kenneth Jamerson, Puja K. Mehta, Erin D. Michos, et al. "Meditation and

Cardiovascular Risk Reduction: A Scientific Statement from the American Heart Association." *Journal of the American Heart Association* 6, no. 10 (September 28, 2017). https://doi.org/10.1161/jaha.117.004176.

Levine, Glenn N., Karen Allen, Lynne T. Braun, Hayley E. Christian, Erika Friedmann, Kathryn A. Taubert, Sue Ann Thomas, Deborah L. Wells, and Richard A. Lange. "Pet Ownership and Cardiovascular Risk." *Circulation* 127, no. 23 (May 9, 2013): 2353–63. https://doi.org/10.1161/cir .0b013e31829201e1.

Lotzof, Kerry. "Are We Really Made of Stardust?" Natural History Museum. Accessed February 27, 2023. https://www.nhm.ac.uk/discover/are-we -really-made-of-stardust.html.

Malhotra, V., R. Bharshankar, N. Ravi, and O. L. Bhagat. "Acute Effects on Heart Rate Variability during Slow Deep Breathing." *Mymensingh Medical Journal* 30, no. 1 (January 2021): 208–13.

Mane, Rekha Vishnu, and Shital Waghmare. "A Study to Assess the Impact of Guided Imagery Therapy on Blood Pressure among Hypertensive Geriatric Group Residing in Selected Old Age Home of Pune City." *International Journal of Health Sciences & Research* 6, no. 7 (July 2016): 228–36.

Marcus, Aubrey. "What." *Aubrey Marcus* (blog), May 9, 2018. https://www .aubreymarcus.com/blogs/poetry/what.

Mariotti, Agnese. "The Effects of Chronic Stress on Health: New Insights into the Molecular Mechanisms of Brain–Body Communication." *Future Science OA* 1, no. 3 (November 2015). https://doi.org/10.4155/fso.15.21.

"Mindfulness Definition: What Is Mindfulness?" Greater Good. Accessed February 22, 2023. https://greatergood.berkeley.edu/topic/mindfulness/ definition.

Mitchell, R. A., and A. J. Berger. "Neural Regulation of Respiration." *American Review of Respiratory Disease* 111, no. 2 (February 1, 1975). https://doi.org /10.1164/arrd.1975.111.2.206.

Monahan, Heather. *Confidence Creator*. Miami, FL: Boss in Heels, 2018.

Morita, E., S. Fukuda, J. Nagano, N. Hamajima, H. Yamamoto, Y. Iwai, T. Nakashima, H. Ohira, and T. Shirakawa. "Psychological Effects of Forest Environments on Healthy Adults: Shinrin-Yoku (Forest-Air Bathing, Walking) as a Possible Method of Stress Reduction." *Public Health* 121, no. 1 (January 2007): 54–63. https://doi.org/10.1016/j.puhe.2006.05.024.

Moszeik, Esther N., Timo von Oertzen, and Karl-Heinz Renner. "Effectiveness of a Short Yoga Nidra Meditation on Stress, Sleep, and Well-Being in a Large and Diverse Sample." *Current Psychology* 41, no. 8 (September 8, 2020): 5272–86. https://doi.org/10.1007/s12144-020-01042-2.

Nemeth, Maria. *Mastering Life's Energies: Simple Steps to a Luminous Life*. Novato, CA: New World Library, 2007.

Ornish, Dean. "Avoiding Revascularization with Lifestyle Changes: The Multicenter Lifestyle Demonstration Project." *American Journal of Cardiology*

82, no. 10 (November 26, 1998): 72–76. https://doi.org/10.1016/s0002
-9149(98)00744-9.

Ornish, Dean, and Anne Ornish. *Undo It!: How Simple Lifestyle Changes Can Reverse Most Chronic Diseases*. New York: Ballantine Books, 2022.

Ornish, Dean, R. J. Brand, C. Hogeboom, R. L. Kirkeeide, T. A. Ports, W. T. Armstrong, S. Sparler, et al. "Intensive Lifestyle Changes for Reversal of Coronary Heart Disease." *JAMA* 280, no. 23 (December 16, 1998): 2001–7. https://doi.org/10.1001/jama.280.23.2001.

Ornish, D., S. E. Brown, J. H. Billings, L. W. Scherwitz, W. T. Armstrong, T. A. Ports, S. M. McLanahan, R. L. Kirkeeide, K. L. Gould, and R. J. Brand. "Can Lifestyle Changes Reverse Coronary Heart Disease?" *The Lancet* 336, no. 8708 (July 22, 1990): 129–33. https://doi.org/10.1016/0140-6736(90)91656-u.

Özlü, Ibrahim, Zeynep Öztürk, Zeynep Karaman Özlü, Erdal Tekin, and Ali Gür. "The Effects of Progressive Muscle Relaxation Exercises on the Anxiety and Sleep Quality of Patients with Covid-19: A Randomized Controlled Study." *Perspectives in Psychiatric Care* 57, no. 4 (March 2, 2021): 1791–97. https://doi.org/10.1111/ppc.12750.

Pal, GopalKrushna, Ankit Agarwal, Shanmugavel Karthik, Pravati Pal, and Nivedita Nanda. "Slow Yogic Breathing through Right and Left Nostril Influences Sympathovagal Balance, Heart Rate Variability, and Cardiovascular Risks in Young Adults." *North American Journal of Medical Sciences* 6, no. 3 (March 2014): 145–51. https://doi.org/10.4103/1947-2714.128477.

Parker, Stephen. "Training Attention for Conscious Non-REM Sleep: The Yogic Practice of Yoga-Nidrā and Its Implications for Neuroscience Research." *Progress in Brain Research*, 2019, 255–72. https://doi.org/10.1016/bs.pbr.2018.10.016.

Perez, Vanessa, Dominik D. Alexander, and William H. Bailey. "Air Ions and Mood Outcomes: A Review and Meta-Analysis." *BMC Psychiatry* 13, no. 1 (January 15, 2013). https://doi.org/10.1186/1471-244x-13-29.

Razani, Nooshin. "Prescribing Nature for Health." *TEDx Talks*. Lecture presented at the TEDx Nashville, June 14, 2016.

Rowden, Adam. "Normal Respiration Rate: For Adults and All Ages, and How to Measure." *Medical News Today*. MediLexicon International, January 4, 2023. https://www.medicalnewstoday.com/articles/324409.

Shmerling, Robert H. "The Placebo Effect: Amazing and Real." *Harvard Health*, June 22, 2020. https://www.health.harvard.edu/blog/the-placebo-effect-amazing-and-real-201511028544.

"Sleep Plays an Important Role in Heart Health." Heart.org, January 13, 2023. https://www.heart.org/en/health-topics/sleep-disorders/sleep-and-heart-health.

Srihari Sharma, K. N., NidhiRam Choudhary, and Pailoor Subramanya. "Evidence Base of Yoga Studies on Cardiovascular Health: A Bibliometric

Analysis." *International Journal of Yoga* 12, no. 2 (May 6, 2019): 162. https: //doi.org/10.4103/ijoy.ijoy_6_18.

Stephens, Rebecca. "Imagery." *Clinical Nurse Specialist* 7, no. 4 (July 1993): 170–74. https://doi.org/10.1097/00002800-199307000-00004.

Sundar, S., S. K. Agrawal, V. P. Singh, S. K. Bhattacharya, K. N. Udupa, and S. K. Vaish. "Role of Yoga in Management of Essential Hypertension." *Acta Cardiologica* 39, no. 3 (January 1, 1984): 203–8.

"The Center for Compassion and Altruism Research: Current Research." The Center for Compassion and Altruism Research and Education. Accessed February 27, 2023. http://ccare.stanford.edu/research/current-research/ #firsttab.

"The Power of Pets." National Institutes of Health. U.S. Department of Health and Human Services, July 26, 2022. https://newsinhealth.nih.gov/2018 /02/power-pets.

"2021–2022 APPA National Pet Owners Survey." American Pet Products Association. Accessed February 27, 2023. https://www.americanpetproducts .org/pubs_survey.asp.

Vonnegut, Kurt. *Mother Night*. London: Vintage Digital, 2020.

"What Causes an Adrenaline Rush? The Impact of Epinephrine and Certain Situations." WebMD, April 27, 2021. https://www.webmd.com/a-to-z -guides/what-to-know-adrenaline-rush.

Index

abdominal breathing (long
breathing), 30, 83–85

activities: for Kapha dosha,
176; for Pitta dosha, 174;
for Vata dosha, 173

adrenal fatigue, 54

adrenal glands, fight or flight
response and, 16, 55, 78, 83,
88, 145

adrenaline stress hormone,
55; shallow breathing and,
78, 83

advice, listening with
compassion and no, 153–54

Ahimsa (non-
harming): animal treatment
and, 147–49; compassion
in, 146–47; kindness in,
147–48; peace and, 147;
respect for all beings in,
147–48

air element: bird-watching
practice, 180–81; kite flying
practice, 181; as Pancha
Maha Bhutas element,
163; practices for, 180–81;

Vata dosha and, 164, 166,
171, 177

alternate nostril breathing,
88–91

American Heart Association,
on meditation, 99

Ana Maya Kosha (food body),
58–59

Ananda Maya Kosha (bliss
body), 61

animals: Ahimsa on kindness
and respect for, 147–48;
pet ownership and, 148–49;
plant-based diet and,
147–48

ankle and feet exercises yoga
warmup, 29, *30*

anxiety: author change with
yoga, 4; imagery to reduce,
133–34, 138

attention, outside of us, 20

automatic breathing, 77

autonomic nervous system,
involuntary actions and, 55

Ayurveda (life wisdom)
system: doshas and, 164–77;

About the Author

Susi Amendola holds both an ERYT 500 with Yoga Alliance and a C-IAYT with the International Association of Yoga Therapists.

As a teenager, Susi began to experience crippling anxiety and depression, and doctors offered little help. One day, her mother took her to a yoga class at a local yoga institute, and Susi experienced an overwhelming sense of calm that she didn't know was possible. Yoga became her refuge, and slowly, she began to find her way back to health.

This experience led her to Pennsylvania, where she became a resident at a yoga institute. There, she spent time working in and managing the vegetarian kitchen while attending daily classes in yoga, meditation, and philosophy. She took workshops in all kinds of health-related topics, ate vegetarian meals, and walked outside in the fresh, open mountain air. The structure, the food, the yoga practices, the sense of community, and living in nature became the foundation and the foothold that Susi needed to find her way back to herself.

After several years of study, work, and practice, she and her new family decided to move to Omaha, Nebraska, to be closer to family. Susi soon founded the Omaha Yoga & Bodywork Center, one of the first and oldest yoga centers in the Midwest. She worked diligently to create programs to train yoga teachers, sponsor well-known speakers on yoga, and bring the healing practices of yoga to businesses, schools, and the community. Today, the center is called Yoga Now, and since its inception in 1983 has served as a stronghold in the community.

In 1993, she joined Ornish Lifestyle Medicine, a Medicare-approved intensive cardiac rehab program, as a stress management specialist and senior trainer. The program includes Yoga and meditation as part of a multidisciplinary approach to healing. For decades, she has traveled extensively to train and mentor hospital teams in delivering this intervention.

As Susi helped others with the practices that turned her own life around, she gathered their stories of health and healing, which served as the inspiration for her teachings and this book. With her expertise in both the ancient practices of Yoga and the medical world, Susi's teachings and classes are unlike anything else you will find. Her teaching style is heart-centered, nurturing, practical, and empowering. She continues to practice, teach, and inspire others to listen deeply to the healer within.

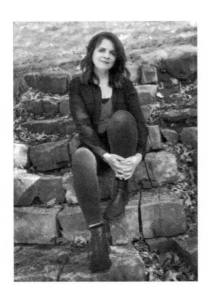